Advanced hairdressing science

Florence Openshaw, B.Sc., M.I.T.

Longman
London and New York

Longman Group Limited
Longman House, Burnt Mill, Harlow
Essex CM20 2JE, England

*Published in the United States of America
by Longman Inc., New York*

First published 1981
Fourth impression 1986

British Library Cataloguing in Publication Data

Openshaw, Florence
 Advanced hairdressing science.
 1. Hairdressing
 I. Title
 646.7'24   TT957
 ISBN 0-582-41583-7

Set in VIP Times Roman 10/11
Produced by Longman Singapore Publishers (Pte) Ltd.
Printed in Singapore.

Contents

Preface

This book is suitable for students studying Hairdressing Science in preparation for the City and Guilds of London Institute Certificate in Advanced Studies in Hairdressing and also for the Manicure Certificate. Whilst the book is complete in itself it assumes a knowledge of the basic science as covered in *Hairdressing Science*, which is intended for students in the early years of their training, and is the forerunner of this book.

The terminology of the book is based on that used in the cosmetic industry and in the hairdressing profession. Chemical names are those used in industry rather than those more acceptable to the pure scientist or used in the teaching of students in pure science. Since all the products entering the salon in bottles, sachets and tubes are labelled in millilitres, the use of cm^3 in the teaching situation seems academic.

The questions at the end of each chapter include both short answer and essay-type. Multiple choice questions are included at the end of the book.

New hairdressing products are constantly being developed, and whilst usually they are suitably labelled for use, in order to understand the various procedures involved hairdressers must have a sound scientific background, whence they can use the products with confidence and also give their clients an accurate explanation of their function. It is therefore hoped that this book will help students to gain a greater understanding of both hair itself and the products used in hairdressing processes.

Acknowledgements

Acknowledgements are due to the following for permission to reproduce illustrations:

Fig 2.1(b) – Microphotograph of section of skin – (Oxford Scientific Films)
Fig 3.2(a) (b) (c) – Bacteria – (C. James Webb)
Fig 3.3 – Influenza viruses – (C. James Webb)
Fig 3.5 – Impetigo – (Institute of Dermatology)
Fig 3.6 – Carbuncle – (Institute of Dermatology)
Fig 3.7 – Herpes simplex – (Institute of Dermatology)
Fig 3.8 – Common wart – (Institute of Dermatology)
Fig 3.10 – Ringworm of the scalp – (C. James Webb)
Fig 3.11(a) (b) – Pediculus capitis & hair clippings – (C. James Webb)
Fig 3.13 – Itch mite – (Institute of Dermatology)
Fig 3.14 – Section showing itch mite – (Institute of Dermatology)
Fig 3.15 – Demodex face mite – (Institute of dermatology)
Fig 3.16 – Common flea – (C. James Webb)
Fig 3.17 – Psoriasis of the scalp – (Institute of Dermatology)
Fig 3.19 – Mole – (Institute of Dermatology)
Fig 3.20 – Skin tags – (Photo Ken Moreman/Vision International)
Fig 3.21 – Contact dermatitis – (Institute of Dermatology)
Fig 3.22 – Acne vulgaris – (Institute of Dermatology)
Fig 4.7 – Micrograph showing cuticle scales – (Wella International)
Fig 4.9 – Transverse section of hair – (L.P.S. Piper, Principal of Cornwall Technical College, Redruth)
Fig 4.10 – Transverse section of hair showing cortex – (L.P.S. Piper, Principal of Cornwall Technical College, Redruth)
Fig 4.17(b) – Structure of cortex – (L.P.S. Piper, Principal of Cornwall Technical College, Redruth)
Fig 4.18 – Micrograph showing cuticle scales and fibres – (Wella International)
Fig 6.1 – Alopecia areata – (Institute of Dermatology)
Fig 6.4 – Traction alopecia – (Wella International)
Fig 7.1 – Structure of an emulsion – (Unilever Educational Publications)
Fig 8.9 – Foam structure – (Unilever Educational Publications)
Fig 8.10 – Detergent acts as wetting agent – (Shell International Petroleum Co. Ltd.)
Fig 8.12 – Detergent action – (Unilever Educational Publications)
Fig 10.11 – How hairspray holds hair (Unilever Research)
Fig 11.3 – Electron micrographs (a) (b) (c) – (L.P.S. Piper, Principal of Cornwall Technical College, Redruth/Central Research Laboratories of the English China Clays Group)
Fig 11.4 – Split end of hair – (Dr Tony Brain/Science Photo Library)
Fig 11.5 – Trichorrhexis nodosa – (Institute of Dermatology)
Fig 12.6 – Ringworm of the nail – (Institute of Dermatology)
Fig 12.7 – Psoriasis causing thimble pitting (Ken Moreman/Vision International)

Chapter 1

The head and neck

The general shape of the head is determined by the formation of the bones of the skull, and by the depth of soft tissue composed of both muscle and subcutaneous fat which lies between the bone and the surface skin. The head contains the brain, the main nerve centre of the body, as well as the sense organs of sight, taste, hearing and smell. The skull provides a rigid structure which protects these delicate organs within the various cavities of the head.

The structure of the skull

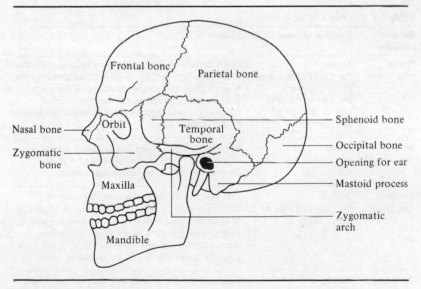

Fig 1.1(a) Side view of the skull

The skull, which consists of twenty-two bones (see Fig. 1.1a and b), may be considered in two parts, the cranium and the face.
The bones of the cranium. The cranium consists of eight bones forming a box-like cavity which holds the brain. The bones of the cranium are listed in Table 1.1.

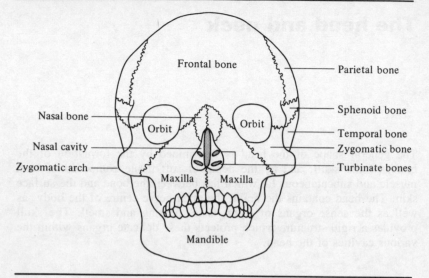

Fig 1.1(b) Front view of the skull

Table 1.1 The bones of the cranium

Bone of cranium	Position of bone	Notes
Frontal (one bone)	Forms: the forehead and front of the cranium, the roof of the orbits, part of the base of the cranium	Contains two large air cavities or sinuses connected to the nasal cavities by small openings, making the bones lighter and giving resonance to the voice. The sinus linings sometimes become infected following a cold. Frontal bone joins parietal bones by the coronal suture
Parietal (two bones)	Forms: the top and sides of the cranium	Regularly shaped bones joining down the mid line •of the skull in the sagittal suture. Also join temporal bones in the squamosal sutures
Occipital (one bone)	Forms: the back and base of the cranium	Contains the foramen magnum, the opening through which the spinal cord passes. A projection or condyle on each side of the opening fits into a corresponding hollow in the first vertebra (the atlas) to allow the head to nod. The occipital bone joins the parietal bones in the lambdoid suture
Temporal (two bones)	Forms: the lower part of the sides of the cranium	Projections from these bones meet the zygomatic bones to form the zygomatic arches on each side of the face. The mastoid processes at the base of the bones jut out just behind the ears and are points of attachment for the sterno-mastoid muscles. The thick lower portion of the bones contain the internal parts of the ears

Bone of cranium	Position of bone	Notes
Sphenoid (one bone)	Forms: most of the base and parts of the sides of the cranium, part of the outer sides of the orbits	Shaped like a bat with its extended wing tips forming part of each side of the skull between the temporal and frontal bones
Ethmoid (one bone)	Forms: part of the orbits, the roof of the nasal cavities, part of the septum or partition between the nostrils	Small irregular shaped bone. The olfactory nerves (nerves of smell) pass through a series of small openings or foramina in this bone

The bones of the face. There are fourteen bones in the face and these are listed in Table 1.2.

Table 1.2 The bones of the face

Bone of face	Position of bone	Notes
Zygomatic or malar (two bones)	Cheek bones, also part of the floor of the orbits	A projection from these bones joins the temporal bones to form the zygomatic arches on each side of the face. The arches form points of attachment for the zygomatic muscles
Maxillae or superior maxillary bones (two bones)	Form the upper jaw and part of the roof of the mouth and the floor of the orbits	These bones hold the upper set of teeth
Mandible or inferior maxillary bone (one bone)	Forms the lower jaw, chin and lower sides of the face	The mandible holds the lower set of teeth. Forms movable joints with the temporal bones to enable chewing and talking to take place
Nasal bones (two bones)	Form the bridge of the nose	The lower part of the nose consists of cartilage which is softer and more flexible than bone. The cartilage determines the shape of the tip of the nose
Lachrymal (two bones)	Form the inner walls of the orbits	Very small bones containing a groove by which lachrymal fluid (tears) passes from the eye to the nasal cavity
Turbinate (two bones)	In the cavity behind the nose	Small scroll-shaped bones over which air flows and is warmed before passing to the lungs

Bone of face	Position of bone	Notes
Palatine (two bones)	In the roof of the mouth forming the back of the hard palate	
Vomer (one bone)	Forms part of the septum between the nostrils	

The joints of the skull

The lower jaw or mandible is attached to the right and left temporal bones by the only movable joints in the skull, to enable chewing and talking to take place. The joints are unusual since they combine hinge and gliding joints to allow a side to side movement as well as an up and down movement of the jaw. The joints between all other bones in the skull are fixed joints called *sutures* which permit no movement (see Fig. 1.2). These bones have saw-like edges which fit accurately together like pieces of a jig-saw puzzle. The main sutures are named in Fig. 1.3 and Fig. 1.4.

At birth the sutures are joined by fibrous tissue so that limited movement of the bones is possible, enabling the baby's head to be moulded slightly during the actual birth. Larger areas of fibrous tissue called *fontanelles* also lie at the junctions of some of the bones and these are not completely closed by bone formation until the child is 12–18 months old. The largest of these areas is the anterior fontanelle between the frontal and parietal bones (see Fig. 1.5). This is often referred to as the soft spot, and a pulse may often be seen beating at this point. Since the area is covered with a sheet of strong fibrous tissue, there is no chance of damage during washing or cutting the child's hair. The closure of the fontanelles leaves the skull rigid with no movement between the bones.

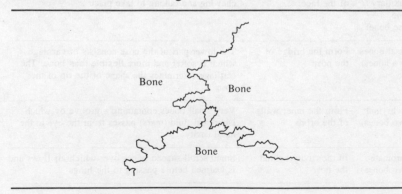

Bone

Bone

Bone

Fig 1.2 Sutures between the bones of the skull

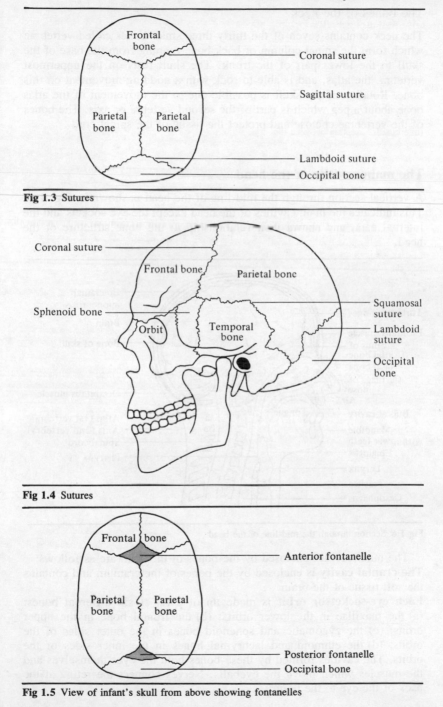

Fig 1.3 Sutures

Fig 1.4 Sutures

Fig 1.5 View of infant's skull from above showing fontanelles

The bones of the neck

The neck contains seven of the thirty-three small bones called vertebrae which form the spinal column or back bone running from the base of the skull to the lower part of the trunk. The skull rests on the uppermost vertebra, the atlas, and is able to rock with a nodding movement on this bone. Rotation of the skull is possible due to the movement of the atlas bone about a peg which is part of the second vertebra or axis. The bones of the vertebrae enclose and protect the tissue of the spinal cord.

The main cavities of the head

A vertical section through the mid-line of the head is shown in Fig. 1.6. This indicates the main cavities of the head except the eye sockets and the internal ears, and shows their relationship to the bone structure of the head.

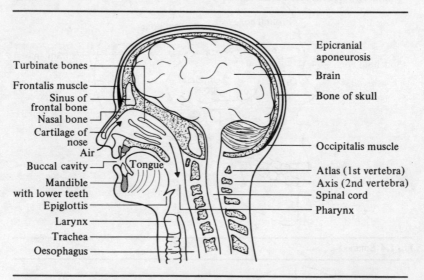

Fig 1.6 Section through the mid-line of the head

The main cavities enclosed by the bones of the skull are as follows:
The cranial cavity is enclosed by the bones of the cranium and contains the soft tissue of the brain.
Each eye-socket or orbit is made up of parts of six different bones: (a) the maxillae in the lower orbits; (b) the frontal bone in the upper orbits; (c) the zygomatic and sphenoid bones in the outer sides of the orbits; (d) the ethmoid and lachrymal bones in the inner sides of the orbits. The cavities formed by these bones hold the eyes themselves and the muscles which move the eyeballs. Nerves connect the retina at the back of the eye to the brain.

The nasal cavities lead from the nostrils to the pharynx. The two cavities are divided by a septum of bone and cartilage. The roof of the cavities is formed by the ethmoid bone through which pass the branches of the olfactory nerve to the brain. Air is forced through the cavities during respiration, the ingoing air being warmed as it passes over the turbinate bones and being moistened by the mucous membranes lining the cavity, before reaching the lungs.

The mouth or buccal cavity is concerned with the intake of food and contains the teeth for mastication, the tongue with its taste buds and the openings of the salivary glands which secrete digestive enzymes into the cavity.

The mouth and nasal cavities are linked at the back of the mouth to form the pharynx or throat which in turn leads to the air and food passages in the neck. The air passage lies at the front of the neck and contains the larynx or voice box (see Fig. 1.6).

The cavity of the ear (the external auditory meatus) is a tunnel about 2 centimetres long leading into the temporal bone. The end of the tunnel is sealed by a membrane, the ear drum, which picks up sounds and transmits them to the middle ear and the inner ear deep in the temporal bone. From the inner ear pulses travel along the auditory nerve to the brain where they give the sensation of sound.

The nervous system of the head and neck

The nervous system consists basically of the brain and the spinal cord with their associated nerves. The spinal cord, an extension of nervous tissue from the brain, passes from the base of the brain through the foramen magnum in the occipital bone, then runs through the bones of the spinal column. These bones protect the soft nerve tissue of the cord. The brain and the spinal cord together make up the *central nervous system*.

One function of the brain is to receive messages via the nerves in the form of electrical impulses generated by the sense organs of the body, that is the eyes, ears, nose, mouth and skin. After interpreting the messages, the brain then sends out impulse signals to the muscles and glands, causing appropriate movements or secretions to take place. The nerves carrying messages into the brain are called *sensory nerves* and those carrying messages from the brain are called *motor nerves* (see Fig. 1.7).

Twelve pairs of nerves are connected directly to the brain and are known as *cranial nerves*. They mostly supply the organs of the head and neck. Thirty-one pairs of nerves are connected directly to the spinal cord and are called *spinal nerves*. Eight of these pairs are connected to the spinal cord in the neck area, and the remainder to the spinal cord in the trunk. The cranial nerves and the spinal nerves together form the *peripheral nervous system*. Impulses passing through these nerves control the voluntary muscles (that is muscles which can be contracted at will), such as the muscles of the limbs and those of facial expression, and also

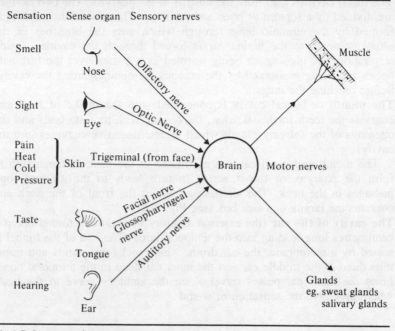

Sensation   Sense organ   Sensory nerves

Smell
Nose
Olfactory nerve

Sight
Eye
Optic Nerve

Pain
Heat
Cold   } Skin   Trigeminal (from face)
Pressure

Taste
Tongue
Facial nerve
Glossopharyngeal nerve

Hearing
Ear
Auditory nerve

Brain   Motor nerves

Muscle

Glands
eg. sweat glands
salivary glands

Fig 1.7 Sensory and motor nerves

supply the skin and other sense organs. Involuntary muscles (which contract automatically without any conscious effort), such as those of the heart and the alimentary tract, are served by another system of nerves known as the *autonomic system*.

When the brain reacts automatically to a sensory stimulus without conscious thought, the action is called a *reflex action*. For example, if an object approaches close to the eyes, blinking of the eyelid automatically takes place. Under certain circumstances, the spinal cord can also react in a similar manner and may pass on messages reflexly without reference to the brain, e.g. if the hand touches a hot object the arm muscles contract to remove the hand immediately (see Fig. 1.8).

In considering the head and neck, the cranial nerves are most important. They serve the sense organs, the muscles and most of the skin of the head. The cranial nerves and their functions are listed in Table 1.3.

The cranial nerves most concerned with the skin and muscles of the face are the fifth and seventh pairs. The eleventh pair or accessory nerves are motor nerves through which the movements of the sternomastoid and trapezius muscles are controlled.

The fifth cranial nerve or trigeminal nerve (see Fig. 1.9) is mainly a sensory nerve which carries information to the brain from the skin of the face, the teeth and the mucous membranes of the nose and mouth. There is a small motor branch to the muscles of mastication. The trigeminal nerve divides into three branches inside the cranium and these pass

Table 1.3 Cranial nerves

Name of nerve	Type	Function and distribution
1. Olfactory nerve	Sensory	Nerve of smell. Carries impulses from the nose to the brain
2. Optic nerve	Sensory	Nerve of sight. Carries impulses from the eye to the brain
3. Oculomotor nerve	Motor	To some of the muscles which move the eyeball and to the eye for constriction of the pupil
4. Trochlear nerve	Motor	To another muscle which moves the eyeball
5. Trigeminal nerve	Motor	To the muscles of mastication.
	Sensory	From the skin of the face, the orbit, the nasal cavity, mouth, teeth and gums
6. Abducent nerve	Motor	To one of the muscles moving the eyeball
7. Facial nerve	Motor	To the muscles of facial expression
	Sensory	Nerve of taste, carries impulses from the front of the tongue
8. Auditory nerve	Sensory	Nerve of hearing and balance. Carries impulses from the ear to the brain
9. Glossopharyngeal nerve	Motor	To the muscles at the back of the throat for swallowing
	Sensory	Nerve of taste from back of tongue
10. Vagus nerve	Motor	To the muscles of respiration, digestive tract, and heart
	Sensory	From the lower pharynx (coughing)
11. Accessory nerve	Motor	To move the sterno-mastoid and trapezius muscles in the neck in bending and turning the head
12. Hypoglossal nerve	Motor	To move the tongue

through different openings or foramina in the sphenoid bone. Each branch has nerve fibres going to the inner part of the face. Some fibres pass through foramina in the facial bones to supply the skin of the face.

The main branches are as follows.

The mandibular branch has both sensory and motor nerve fibres. It is sensory to the teeth of the lower jaw, the mucous membranes of the mouth and cheeks, and the skin of the lower and back part of the face. The motor fibres lead to the masseter and temporalis muscles, the muscles of mastication.

The maxillary branch is purely sensory and serves the upper jaw, the mucous membranes of the pharynx and the skin on the temples, sides of the forehead and the upper cheeks.

The ophthalmic branch is also sensory and supplies the tear glands, and the skin of the forehead, nose and upper eyelids.

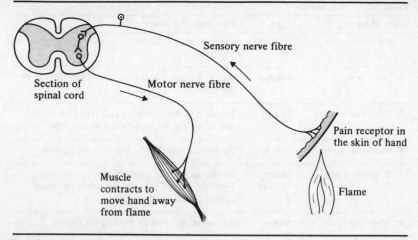

Fig 1.8 Reflex action

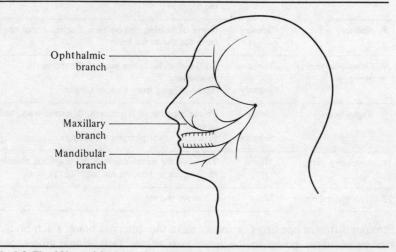

Fig 1.9 The fifth cranial nerve – the trigeminal nerve

The areas of skin served by each branch are shown in Fig. 1.10.

The skin at the back of the head is supplied by the spinal nerves in the neck.

The seventh cranial nerve or the facial nerve is mainly a motor nerve serving the muscles of facial expression, but has a small sensory section for the sensation of taste from the front of the tongue. The nerve passes from the cranium through a foramen in the temporal bone behind the ear, and after a division leading to one of the ear muscles and the occipitalis at the back of the head, the main nerve branches into five parts to the various muscles of the face.

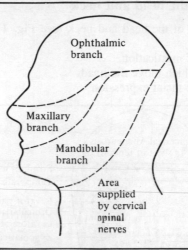

Fig 1.10 Areas of the skin supplied by the trigeminal nerve

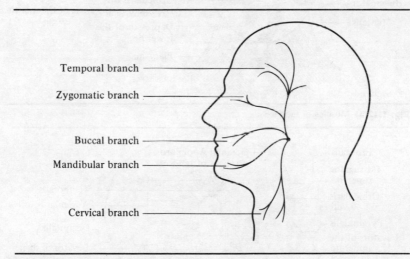

Fig 1.11 The seventh cranial nerve – the facial nerve

The branches (see Fig. 1.11) are as follows.

The temporal branch leads to the auricular muscles behind the ears, the orbicularis oculi and the frontalis muscle.

The zygomatic branch supplies the orbicularis oculi.

The buccal branch goes to the buccinator, the upper lip, the risorius muscle and the side of the nose.

The mandibular branch serves the lower lip and mentalis muscle.

The cervical branch supplies the platysma muscle in the neck.

The muscles of the head and neck

The chief muscles of the head and neck (see Fig. 1.12a and b) fall into three groups.
1. The muscles of mastication.
2. The muscles which move the head.
3. The muscles of facial expression.

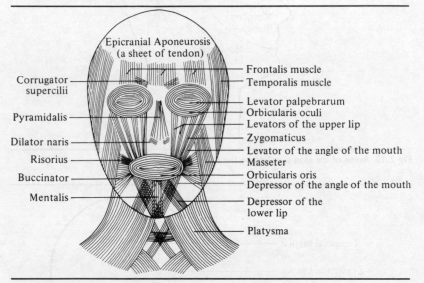

Corrugator supercilii
Pyramidalis
Dilator naris
Risorius
Buccinator
Mentalis

Epicranial Aponeurosis (a sheet of tendon)

Frontalis muscle
Temporalis muscle
Levator palpebrarum
Orbicularis oculi
Levators of the upper lip
Zygomaticus
Levator of the angle of the mouth
Masseter
Orbicularis oris
Depressor of the angle of the mouth
Depressor of the lower lip
Platysma

Fig. 1.12(a) Muscles of the face

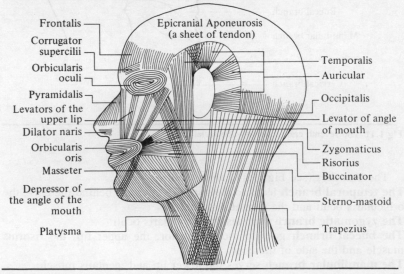

Frontalis
Corrugator supercilii
Orbicularis oculi
Pyramidalis
Levators of the upper lip
Dilator naris
Orbicularis oris
Masseter
Depressor of the angle of the mouth
Platysma

Epicranial Aponeurosis (a sheet of tendon)

Temporalis
Auricular
Occipitalis
Levator of angle of mouth
Zygomaticus
Risorius
Buccinator
Sterno-mastoid
Trapezius

Fig. 1.12(b) Muscles of the head and neck

Muscles form the flesh which covers the bones of the skull. These are all voluntary muscles, being under the control of the will. Each muscle consists of bundles of contractile fibres enclosed in a sheath of fibrous tissue which narrows towards the ends of the muscles to form the tendon attaching the muscle to the bone or to the skin. Contraction of the muscle fibres results in movement of the bone or skin. For example, the lower jaw is raised by the contraction of the muscles of mastication, and the wrinkling of the skin in frowning is caused by the contraction of the supercilii muscles in the forehead.

The contraction of muscles depends on nerve impulses from the brain. Supplies of glucose and oxygen are also necessary to provide energy for contraction and these are brought to the muscle by the arterial blood system. Thus muscles always require an adequate blood and nerve supply (see Fig. 1.13). The point at which the nerve enters the muscle fibres is known as the *motor point* and it is at this point that contraction of the muscle is stimulated during electrical massage.

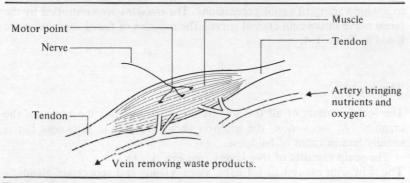

Fig. 1.13 Blood and nerve supply to a muscle

The muscles of mastication

The masseter and temporalis muscles are the chief muscles of mastication. Movement of these muscles is brought about by the action of the trigeminal nerve (fifth cranial nerve). The masseters extend from the zygomatic arch to the angle of the lower jaw. Contraction of the muscles raises the lower jaw and clenches the teeth. The temporalis muscles are fan-shaped and extend from the temporal bone to the lower jaw. Contraction of the temporalis muscles raises the jaw, draws it backwards if protruding, and allows the jaw to move from side to side in grinding movements.

The muscles which move the head

The sternomastoid muscles and trapezius muscles are responsible for head movements. They are controlled by the accessory nerve (eleventh cranial nerve). The sternomastoid muscles extend from the breast bone or sternum, to the mastoid process which is part of the temporal bone and is situated just behind the ears. The muscles thus pass one on each side of the neck. When both the muscles contract together the head moves down as in nodding. When used singly the head is turned to the side opposite to the contracting muscle.

The trapezius muscles are broad flat muscles extending from the occipital bone at the back of the skull to the shoulder blades, and thus cover the back of the neck. The two muscles acting together draw the head backwards. Contraction of one of the muscles only, draws the head to the side of the contracting muscle. These muscles may also be used to raise the shoulders.

The muscles of facial expression

Many muscles concerned with facial expression are attached at both ends to skin rather than bone. On contraction they wrinkle the skin, giving rise to a wide variety of facial expressions. The muscles are controlled by the facial nerve or seventh cranial nerve. The muscles of facial expression are listed in Table 1.4.

The scalp

The scalp consists of all the soft tissue which overlies the bones of the cranium. At the vertex, the scalp is about 5.0 mm in thickness but is usually less in cases of baldness.

The scalp consists of five layers (see Fig. 1.14).
The skin with many hair follicles, sweat glands and sebaceous glands.

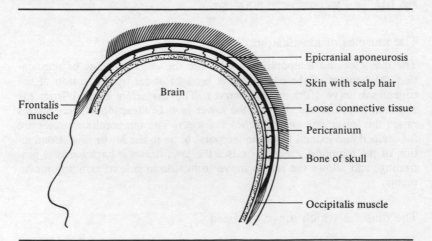

Fig. 1.14 The scalp

Table 1.4 The muscles of facial expression

Group	Name of muscle	Position	Action
Muscles of lips and cheeks	Orbicularis oris	Circular muscle round the mouth.	Closes the mouth. Also used in whistling and pouting
	Risorius	Radiates from the corner of the mouth	Causes smiling
	Buccinator	Inside cheeks.	Keeps food between teeth during mastication. Puffs out the cheeks as in blowing
	Levator of upper lip	Radiates from upper lip	Raises upper lip
	Zygomaticus	Radiates from upper lip	Raises upper lip
	Levator of angle of mouth	Radiates from upper lip	Raises the corners of the mouth
	Depressor of lower lip	Radiates from lower lip	Draws down lower lip
	Depressor of the angle of the mouth	Radiates from lower lip	Draws down the corner of the mouth
	Mentalis	Radiates from lower lip	Turns lower lip outwards
Muscles of forehead	Frontalis	Attached to the epicranial aponeurosis	Wrinkles forehead horizontally and moves the scalp
	Corrugator supercilii	Small muscle under eyebrow	Vertical wrinkles in forehead (frowning)
Muscles of eye area	Orbicularis oculi	Circular muscle round eye	Closes eyelids
	Levator palpebrae	In upper eyelids	Opens upper eyelids
Muscles of ears	Auricular muscles	Group of three muscles above and behind the ears	Move ears slightly (in some people)
Muscles of nose	Pyramidalis	On front of nose	Wrinkles nose
	Dilator naris	At the side of the nostrils	Dilates the nostrils
Muscles of neck	Platysma	Sheet of muscle just under the skin of the neck	Used in expressing sudden fear or when looking fierce

The subcutaneous layer of fatty tissue with a large quantity of fibrous tissue which binds it firmly to the layer below. The main arteries to the skin pass through this layer, forming a network parallel to the surface of the skin, with branches carrying an abundant supply of blood directly to the skin.

The epicranial aponeurosis, a sheet of fibrous tissue or tendon, which extends over the top of the head from the forehead to the back of the head. At the forehead it is connected to the frontalis muscle and at the back of the head to the occipitalis muscle.

Loose connective tissue holds the epicranial aponeurosis to the pericranium. This enables the first three layers, which are closely bound together, to move as one structure over the bones of the skull during massage of the scalp or during shampooing. The looseness of this tissue means that the scalp is easily stripped off by accident, for instance if the hair is caught in machinery.

The pericranium, a thin skin covering the bones of the skull.

The blood supply to the head and neck

All parts of the head and neck including the muscles of the face, skin, scalp, brain and other internal parts receive oxygenated blood supplied by the *carotid arteries*. The left common carotid artery branches from the aorta soon after it leaves the heart, whilst the right common carotid artery branches from the right subclavian artery as shown in Fig. 1.15. The two common carotids then pass one on either side of the trachea in the neck, until at about the level of the Adam's apple they each divide into an

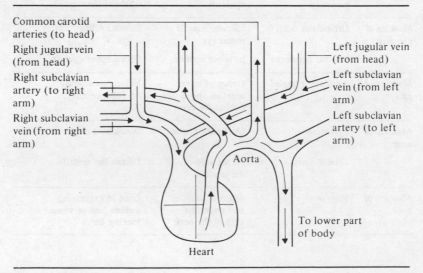

Common carotid arteries (to head)
Right jugular vein (from head)
Right subclavian artery (to right arm)
Right subclavian vein (from right arm)
Left jugular vein (from head)
Left subclavian vein (from left arm)
Left subclavian artery (to left arm)
Aorta
To lower part of body
Heart

Fig 1.15 The common carotid arteries

internal and an external branch. The internal carotid arteries enter the cranium by foramina in the temporal bones just behind the ears and supply the brain, eyes and internal ears.

The external carotid arteries remain outside the skull and supply the muscles of the face, scalp and skin of the head, each artery dividing into three main branches (see Fig. 1.16).

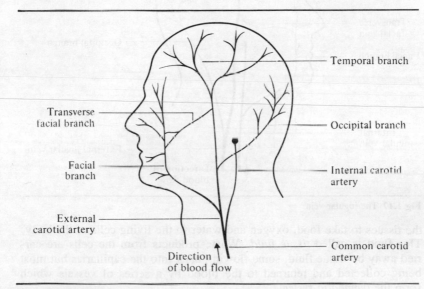

Fig 1.16 The carotid artery

The occipital branch on each side supplies the skin at the back of the head and the scalp as far as the vertex, the two branches joining each other and the temporal branch, to form a network over the scalp.

The temporal branch on each side passes up the side of the face just in front of the ear, subdividing above the surface of the epicranial aponeurosis to feed the capillary networks of the skin including the hair follicles at the top and sides of the head.

The facial branch on each side takes blood to the muscles and skin of the face and joins the temporal branches by the tranverse facial arteries.

De-oxygenated blood in the capillaries of the head and neck collects into the branches of the *jugular veins* which pass down each side of the neck and return blood to the heart via the superior vena cava (see Fig. 1.17).

The lymphatic system of the head and neck

Blood is normally contained in a closed system of blood vessels and does not come into direct contact with the body cells. However, a fluid similar to blood plasma seeps through the capillary walls and circulates through

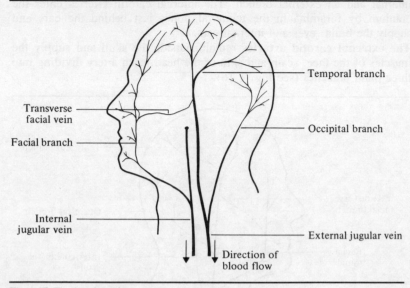

Fig 1.17 The jugular vein

the tissues to take food, oxygen and water to the living cells of the body. This fluid is called *tissue fluid*. Waste products from the cells are carried away by tissue fluid, some flowing back into the capillaries but most being collected and returned to the blood by a series of vessels which form the *lymphatic system*.

The smallest lymph vessels arise in the tissues as blind tubes and form a network which unites into larger lymph vessels. The fluid in these

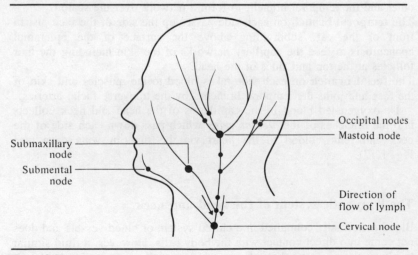

Fig 1.18 The lymph drainage of the head

vessels is known as *lymph*. It is forced along by movement of the surrounding muscles and is prevented from flowing backwards by pocket valves in the walls of the vessels.

At certain points along the vessels are *lymph nodes* (see Fig. 1.18) about the size of a pea, which act as filters for the removal of bacteria. If the tissues are infected the nodes may become swollen and tender, a condition commonly known as swollen glands. If the infection is slight the bacteria are overcome by white blood cells in the node. If the infection is severe there may be acute inflammation of the node and white cells may be destroyed, forming pus which causes an abscess in the node. Lymph from the front of the face, the mouth and tongue is filtered through the submaxillary nodes in the chin. At the lower back of the head, the occipital nodes may become swollen if a septic condition occurs on the back of the head. Further groups of nodes, the cervical nodes, are situated in the neck.

The lymphatic vessels eventually empty the lymph back into the blood system via the subclavian veins near the heart.

Questions

1. What is meant by tissue fluid?
   Describe its main functions.
2. Explain why a septic condition on the back of the scalp is often accompanied by a small swelling in the back of the neck.
3. What are the functions of the:
   (a) internal carotid artery;   (b) external carotid artery;
   (c) jugular vein?
4. What is meant by:
   (a) a motor point;   (b) a motor nerve;   (c) a voluntary muscle?
5. Name three muscles responsible for facial expression and state the function of each.
6. Explain the meaning of each of the following:
   (a) a reflex action;   (b) sinuses;   (c) foramina;   (d) cranial nerves;   (e) a mucous membrane.
   Give an example in each case.
7. Discuss the functions of the skull.
8. Explain what is meant by the sense organs of the head. Along which nerves are impulses transmitted from each of the sense organs to the brain?
9. Explain the action of the muscles which:
   (a) move the head;   (b) move the scalp forwards and backwards;   (c) close the mouth.
   Which nerves control these muscles?
10. What are the functions of the lymphatic system?
    Describe the lymph drainage of the head.

Chapter 2

The skin

The skin forms a flexible covering over the entire surface of the body, though there are considerable variations in the skin of different areas. In some parts of the body, such as the soles of the feet and the palms of the hands, the skin is thick, whilst on the lips, the inner surfaces of the limbs and the abdomen it is much thinner. There are areas of *glabrous* (hairless) skin, areas covered with fine downy hair and others with coarse terminal type hair. The degree of greasiness also varies and depends on the presence and activity of the sebaceous glands in the area. The colour too may vary, not only between different people and different races, but also in different parts of the same body.

The structure of the skin

A section of the general structure of the skin is shown in Fig. 2.1.

The skin is divided into two main layers:

The epidermis (cuticle or scarf skin) forms the outer layer.

The dermis (cutis vera or corium) forms the inner layer and the main bulk of the skin.

Below the dermis is the fatty subcutaneous layer which in most parts of the body, including the face, loosely attaches the skin to the underlying muscles. In the case of the scalp area there is no underlying muscle and the subcutaneous layer lies between the dermis and the epicranial aponeurosis (a sheet of fibrous tissue or tendon) and attaches the two structures firmly together.

The various appendages of the skin, the hair follicles containing the growing hairs, the nails, the sweat glands and the sebaceous glands, are all modifications of epidermal tissue although they appear to be part of the dermis.

The epidermis

The thickness of the epidermis varies in different parts of the body from about 0.1 mm to 2 mm, being thin in the eyelids and abdomen and thickest on the soles of the feet and the palms of the hands. The epidermis consists of five layers of cells though there are no sharp divisions between the layers. The outer layer of flat dead scaly cells is composed of the

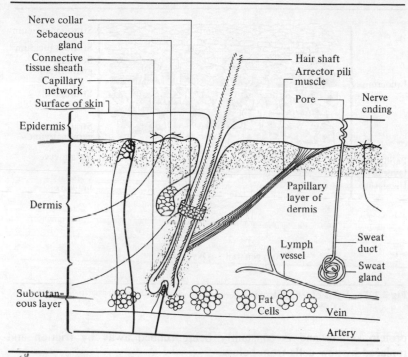

Nerve collar
Sebaceous gland
Connective tissue sheath
Capillary network
Surface of skin
Epidermis
Dermis
Subcutaneous layer

Hair shaft
Arrector pili muscle
Pore
Nerve ending
Papillary layer of dermis
Lymph vessel
Sweat duct
Sweat gland
Fat Cells
Vein
Artery

Fig. 2.1(a) Section of the skin

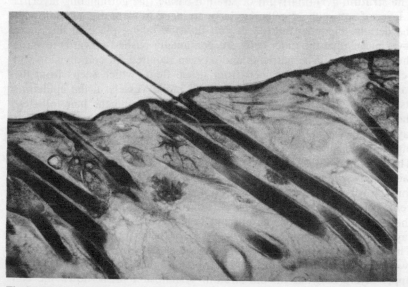

Fig 2.1(b) Microphotograph of section of skin

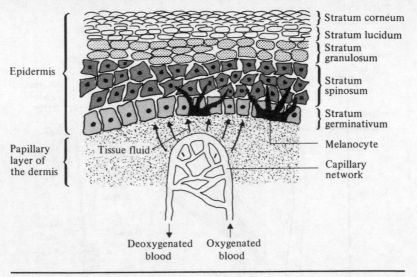

Fig 2.2 The layers of the epidermis

protein keratin and is constantly being rubbed away by friction and replaced by new cells from below.

The layers of the epidermis are shown in Fig. 2.2. Starting with the lowest layer they are as follows:

The stratum germinativum or stratum basale (the germinating layer) is a layer of soft, cuboid cells regularly arranged to form the junction with the dermis. Frequent mitosis or cell division taking place in this basal layer means that the older cells are continually pushed upwards towards the skin surface. The nutrients and oxygen required for cell division and cell development are obtained from tissue fluid, which seeps from the capillaries in the dermis as there are no blood vessels in the epidermis itself. The stratum germinativum is continuous round the hair follicles, the sweat glands and the sebaceous glands. Amongst the cells of this layer are special cells called *melanocytes*, which produce granules of the pigment melanin to give colour to the skin.

The stratum spinosum or stratum aculeatum (the prickle cell layer) contains cells which develop spiny outgrowths or intercellular bridges, through which it is thought that granules of melanin pass into the prickle cells from the melanocytes. The two lower layers of the epidermis form the living part of the epidermis and together are called the Malpighian layer or rete mucosum.

The stratum granulosum (the granular layer) forms the transition between the living cells of the lower layers and the dead scaly cells of the upper layer. Enzymes in the stratum granulosum break down the cell nuclei leading to the death of the cells, the spines become less distinct and the production of keratin begins by the formation of keratohyalin granules. The cells become harder and flatter.

The stratum lucidum (the clear layer) is very shallow in the face, but is thick in the skin of the soles of the feet and the palms of the hands. The flattened cells of this layer are completely filled with keratin. They have no nuclei and the melanin granules have been destroyed by enzymes.

The stratum corneum (the horny layer) is the outer layer of the epidermis and consists of flat hard keratin scales which are gradually shed from the surface of the skin by friction. All epidermal cells are replaced approximately once a month, and in adults about 20 per cent of the dietary intake of protein is used in the constant replacement of skin, hair and nails.

The dermis

The dermis has an average thickness of 3 mm and may be divided into two layers though there is no sharp division between the two.

The papillary layer or upper layer joins the epidermis in a series of ridges called the *dermal papillae*. The layer is continuous round the hair follicles forming a *connective tissue sheath* round each follicle. The dermal papillae each contain a network of blood capillaries. The papillary layer consists of bundles of white non-elastic fibres of the protein, collagen and some yellow elastic fibres both embedded in a jelly-like ground substance.

The reticular layer lies below the papillary layer, and contains a dense network of collagen fibres mostly in layers, which lie parallel to the skin surface with alternate layers at right angles to each other. Between the collagen fibres are loosely woven networks of elastic fibres which enable the skin to stretch, for example in pregnancy or in mumps, and to spring back when released. The jelly like ground substance of mucopolysaccharides absorbs a considerable amount of water, making the skin turgid.

The cells of the dermis
Amongst the fibres of the dermis there are three types of cells.

Mast cells secrete histamine when the skin is damaged, so causing dilation of the blood vessels which brings extra blood to the area to aid repair.

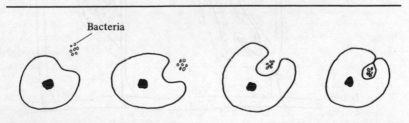

Fig 2.3 Phagocytic cell destroying bacteria

Phagocytic cells are wandering white blood cells which surround and digest foreign matter or bacteria which have entered the skin. The cytoplasm of these cells changes shape, enabling the cells to move and enclose the bacteria (see Fig. 2.3).

Fibroblasts are concerned with the secretion of mucopolysaccharides for the ground substance of the dermis and also play a part in the production of collagen fibres.

The dermis contains several networks of blood vessels, lymph vessels and nerves. The boundary between the dermis and epidermis is clearly defined but the dermis gradually merges with the subcutaneous layer below.

The blood supply to the skin

The dermis is well supplied with blood vessels, partly to supply nutrients to the actively dividing cells of the epidermis to which there is no direct supply, but also to enable the skin to play its part in the regulation of body temperature. A network or plexus of arteries in the subcutaneous layer or the lower dermis runs parallel to the skin's surface. Smaller vessels leave the *dermal plexus* at right angles extending towards the surface of the skin, with branches leading off to form capillary networks round the hair follicles, sweat glands and sebaceous glands (see Fig. 2.4).

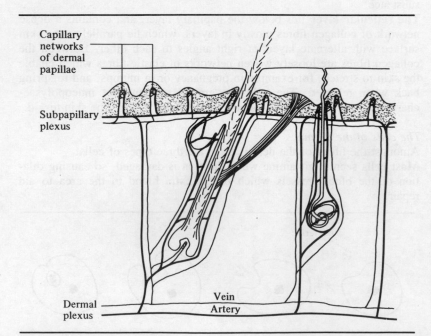

Capillary networks of dermal papillae

Subpapillary plexus

Vein
Artery

Dermal plexus

Fig 2.4 Blood supply to the skin

These smaller vessels join to form another plexus just below the papillary layer of the dermis (*the sub-papillary plexus*). Branches from this second plexus form capillary networks in the dermal papillae just below the epidermis. De-oxygenated blood passes back through a series of small veins to the main venous network of the skin in the lower dermis.

The amount of blood flowing near the surface of the skin is controlled by nerve endings in the artery walls. If the body is becoming overheated, perhaps by exercise or by working in a hot salon, the small skin arteries become dilated, increasing the blood flow to the skin. This causes flushing of the skin, and increases the heat lost from the skin by convection currents set up in the surrounding air, and also by radiation and conduction from the skin. If the body is cooled due to the low temperature of the surrounding air, the small arteries are constricted, less blood flows near the surface of the skin and therefore less heat is lost. The rapid changes required in the blood supply to the skin are possible due to the many alternative pathways or *anastomoses* for the blood at various levels in the skin.

The nerves of the skin

The nerves of the skin are mostly sensory nerves, their function being to detect changes in the outside environment of the body and to relay the information to the brain. The dermis has two main networks of nerves both lying roughly parallel to the skin's surface, one just below the epidermis and the other in the lower dermis. Branches from both have nerve endings of different types detecting cold, heat, pain and pressure. Most of the endings lie in the dermis but a few branched nerve endings which detect pain enter the lower layers of the epidermis (see Fig. 2.5).

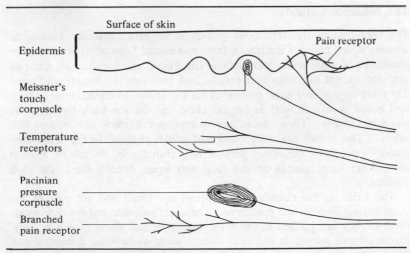

Fig 2.5 Nerve endings in glabrous skin

The nerves of touch or pressure end in rounded touch corpuscles either as Meissners corpuscles, found mostly in the dermal papillae of the finger tips, or Pacinian corpuscles, which lie deep in the dermis of glabrous skin and are sensitive to strong pressure on the skin. In hairy skin the nerves of touch and pain have free branched endings including a collar of nerves round the follicles which is stimulated by light touch of the hairs. Changes of temperature are detected by special endings sensitive to heat and cold.

Motor nerves in the skin include those responsible for the dilation of the blood vessels, the secretion of sweat and the raising of hairs by contraction of the arrector pili muscles.

The glands of the skin

A gland is an organ which takes materials from the blood and manufactures from them a new substance or group of substances which pass out of the gland as a *secretion*. The gland may have a duct or passage along which the secretion flows, or the secretion may enter the blood stream directly from the gland in which case it is known as a ductless gland or *endocrine gland*.

The glands of the skin, the sweat glands and sebaceous glands, pass their secretions through ducts to form a coating on the surface of the skin which is often referred to as the *acid mantle*, since the secretions have a pH of between 4.5 and 6. The acid mantle may be temporarily neutralised by alkali when the skin is washed with soap, but this has no lasting effect as the soap is quickly rinsed away and the acid mantle is restored by further secretion from the glands.

The sebaceous glands

The secretion of the sebaceous glands is an oily substance known as *sebum*, which consists mainly of fats, waxes and fatty acids with smaller quantities of many other substances. The glands are found in all areas of the skin except the soles and palms, and between the fingers and toes. They are largest and most numerous on the scalp, forehead, nose, cheek and beard areas, as well as on the chest and on the back between the shoulder blades. These areas are sometimes known as 'seborrhoeic areas'. The glands are multilobed and pouch shaped. In the scalp they usually open into the upper part of hair follicles by means of a short duct. Very large glands on the face may open directly on to the skin surface.

The cells on the outside of the gland are small and are part of the germinating layer of the epidermis. These cells divide and become modified as they are pushed towards the centre of the gland (see Fig. 2.6). Production of sebum in the cells causes them to become distended and filled with oil when mature. The largest cells at the centre of the gland

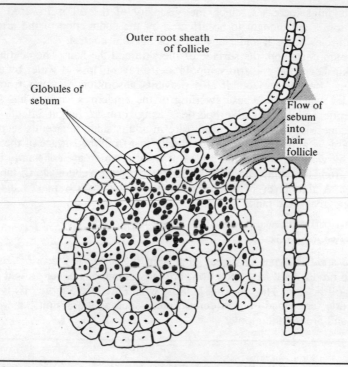

Outer root sheath of follicle

Globules of sebum

Flow of sebum into hair follicle

Fig 2.6 Production of sebum in a sebaceous gland

break down first, the whole cell disintegrating and being discharged with the sebum. This type of secretion which involves the breakdown of the secreting cell itself is termed a *holocrine secretion*. The loss of cells from the centre of the gland is balanced by the production of new cells at the outer edge of the gland.

The secretion of sebum is continuous and depends on the size of the gland, the size being regulated by *hormones* (chemicals secreted directly into the blood from endocrine glands). Male sex hormones increase the size of the glands and therefore the amount of secretion, whereas female sex hormones reduce the size, thus decreasing the secretion. At puberty, increased secretion of the hormone testosterone causes enlargement of the glands, increasing sebum production which often leads to cases of acne at that time. Hormone changes in pregnancy cause reduced sebaceous activity whilst some oral contraceptives cause increased sebum production. In women, hormonal changes at the menopause result in reduced secretion but in older males sufficient testosterone is produced to maintain sebaceous secretion so no corresponding change takes place. Male pattern baldness is also linked with high hormone secretion, so bald heads are often shiny with the sebum produced from enlarged sebaceous glands.

The flow of sebum may also be increased if the temperature of the surroundings increases, since the viscosity of the oil is lowered. The secretion is not thought to be affected by the contraction of the arrector pili muscles nor is it under any form of nervous control.

Sebum coats both the surface of the skin and the hair. The coating on the skin keeps the epidermis supple as it prevents loss of water by evaporation from the surface. It also prevents absorption of water from the outside, which could cause swelling of the epidermis. Sebum has slight antiseptic and fungicidal properties. Ringworm, a fungal infection, is commonest amongst children but rare in adults since sebaceous secretion increases at puberty. Sebum is gradually lost from the surface of the skin, both by washing and on the scales of keratin which are constantly being shed from the skin. Brushing helps to distribute sebum along the hair shafts. A thin layer of sebum adds lustre, but excess makes the hair appear greasy and lank.

The sweat glands

There are two types of sweat glands in the skin. The eccrine glands, which produce a watery secretion, are most numerous being present in all areas of the skin. The apocrine glands, which produce a more oily type of secretion, are found only in certain areas such as the armpits, the pubic area and around the nipples.

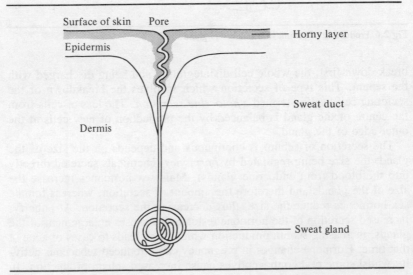

Fig 2.7 An eccrine sweat gland

Eccrine sweat glands or suderiferous glands (see Fig. 2.7) are formed about the fourth foetal month as tubular downgrowths of the germinating layer of the epidermis into the dermis. The number of glands is fixed at birth, so the density of glands decreases as the area of the skin increases during body growth. The glands are most numerous in the areas of the soles of the feet and the palms of the hands.

Sweat glands consist of a coiled tube lying in the dermis, with a duct which is straight at first but takes a spiral course through the epidermis to open in a pore on the skin surface. The spiral structure allows for the distortion of the skin by pressure exerted on its surface.

Sweat is a clear liquid containing 98 per cent water with 2 per cent of sodium chloride and traces of many other substances including urea and lactic acid. The main function of sweat is to help to maintain constant body temperature by cooling the skin. The evaporation of sweat requires latent heat which is taken from the skin, so cooling the body. Continual sweating (insensible perspiration) takes place in temperate climates at the rate of about one litre a day without the skin becoming wet. Secretion of sweat is increased by heat and nervous tension. Excessive perspiration, for example due to extreme physical activity, may cause severe loss of salt from the body resulting in muscular cramp.

The glands are well supplied with blood vessels. A network of capillaries surrounds the gland itself, and two or three capillaries run the length of the duct in the dermis with some cross vessels between them. The capillaries join the network of the subpapillary plexus. The blood supply to the glands remains unchanged even in old age and the working of the glands is continuous throughout life.

The apocrine sweat glands or odoriferous glands (see Fig. 2.8) consist of coiled tubes which are larger than those of the eccrine glands. The

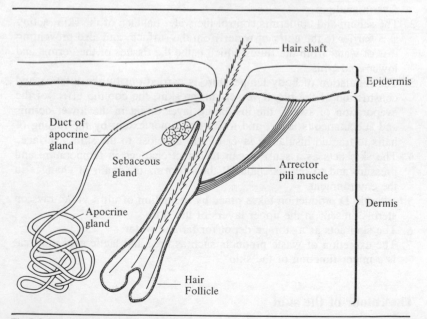

Fig 2.8 Hair follicle with apocrine gland

glands are associated with hair follicles and are limited to certain areas such as the pubic area and the axillae (armpits). They open into the hair follicles above the level of the sebaceous glands or directly on to the surface of the skin near a follicle opening. Development of the glands takes place at puberty, the secretion being under hormonal control as well as nervous control. The secretion is a milky emulsion containing fat particles and the breakdown of this type of perspiration by bacteria leads to unpleasant body odours.

The functions of the skin

1. The skin protects the body from dirt, minor injuries, bacterial invasion and chemical attack. The first barrier is the acid mantle, the acidity (pH 4.5–6) discouraging bacterial growth and the fungicidal properties of sebum preventing fungal growth. The second barrier is the stratum corneum which acts as a filter for invading organisms. The continuity of protection is ensured as damage to the skin is quickly repaired by the multiplication of the cells of the basal layer. The epidermal cells of the outer root sheath and the sweat ducts are also capable of modification for this purpose. If the invading substances pass through the barrier to the lower living layers they diffuse through the cells more easily but may be attacked and removed in the dermis by wandering phagocytic white blood cells. The presence of melanin in the skin protects the underlying tissue from damage by ultra-violet rays in sunlight.
2. The sebum and epidermis control the water balance of the skin, acting as a barrier to the entry of water from the surface, and also preventing loss of water from the fluids which bathe the tissues of the dermis and lower epidermis.
3. The regulation of body temperature is carried out by the dilation and constriction of the blood vessels in the skin, the cooling effect of the evaporation of sweat, the insulating layer of fat in the lower dermis and subcutaneous layer, and to a very minor extent by the raising of hairs to trap an insulating layer of still air close to the skin's surface.
4. The skin acts as a sense organ to detect changes in temperature and pressure and to register pain. It thus informs the brain of changes in the environment.
5. Vitamin D production takes place by the action of ultra-violet rays on sterols present in the upper layers of the skin.
6. The skin acts as a storage depot for fat and water.
7. The excretion of waste products such as urea and lactic acid in sweat is a minor function of the skin.

The colour of the skin

Amongst the cells of the germinating layer of the epidermis are a number of melanocytes which do not divide or travel to the surface of the skin as do the normal basal cells. Their function is to produce granules containing the pigment melanin, and to distribute the granules to the cells of the prickle cell layer by means of *intercellular bridges* or *dendrites* which protrude from the cells (see Fig. 2.9). Each melanocyte is in contact with about ten epidermal cells.

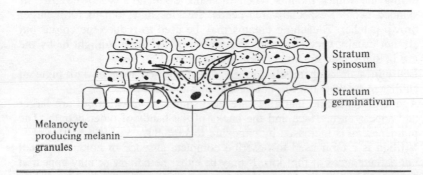

Fig 2.9 Transfer of melanin granules

Melanin itself is formed in the melanocytes by the oxidation of the amino acid *tyrosine*, under the influence of an enzyme called *tyrosinase*. The amount of melanin produced is affected by hormones which are secreted by the pituitary gland at the base of the brain and by the secretion of the adrenal glands.

The function of melanin is to absorb harmful ultra-violet rays from the sun which could cause inflammation and blisters if they reached the papillary layer of the dermis. In white races, melanin is normally broken down through enzyme action by the time it reaches the stratum lucidum. Exposure to ultra-violet rays, however, prevents this breakdown causing darkening of the melanin and stimulating the melanocytes to increase melanin production. The actual number of melanocytes is not increased. In dark skinned races, the melanocytes are more active and produce greater quantities of melanin although the actual number of melanocytes may be no greater than in white races. The rate of removal of melanin as the cells move towards the skin surface is also less.

The final colour of the skin depends on:
1. The amount of melanin produced.
2. The amount of pigment removed by enzyme action.
3. The natural yellowish colour (carotene) of the epidermal cells themselves.
4. The amount of blood flowing through the capillaries of the upper dermis. If the blood vessels are dilated, the skin becomes red due to oxyhaemoglobin in the red blood cells. If the vessels are constricted by cold, the blood flow is slower and the presence of de-oxygenated blood makes the skin blue.

Variation in normal colour

Freckles (ephelides) are due to localised collections of pigment which are unevenly distributed in the stratum germinativum. They only appear on surfaces of the skin which have been exposed to sunlight, the production of melanin being stimulated by ultra-violet rays. Freckles tend to fade during the winter months when melanin production is slowed. In fair skinned people, especially red-heads, freckles may join to form larger brown patches. Bleaching creams may be used to reduce the colour but are not usually very effective. Prevention by avoiding sunlight or by the use of sun-screen creams is more satisfactory.

Lentigines are congenitally formed, slightly raised areas of dark pigment similar to freckles but are unaffected by sunlight.

Age spots or senile lentigines are also similar to freckles but are larger and appear on the face and the backs of the hands of older people. The pigmentation is increased by exposure to sunlight.

Vitiligo is a term used to describe complete absence of colour in small but definite areas of the skin. It may be either hereditary or may appear at any age. The skin is of normal texture and the condition is best treated by cosmetic camouflage.

Albinism is a congenital defect in which melanocytes are present but inactive. No pigment is produced anywhere in the body so that the hair and skin are white and there is no colour in the iris of the eyes. The condition is due to an enzyme disorder in which no tyrosinase is manufactured by the cells. A person suffering from this defect is known as an albino.

The effect of ultra-violet rays on the skin

Ultra-violet rays are present in sunlight but may also be produced artificially by a carbon arc or by a mercury vapour lamp. Ultra-violet treatment is now offered by many salons to produce tanning of the skin. Treatment by ultra-violet rays is also useful in cases of psoriasis and acne. The rays form part of the electromagnetic spectrum (see Fig. 2.10). Ultra-violet rays have the following effect on the skin:

1. The rays are absorbed by the skin, the most active being in one particular band of wavelengths (290–320 nanometres). Mild exposure to

X-rays	Visible light			
	Ultra-violet rays	Infra-red rays	Radio waves

Fig 2.10 The electromagnetic spectrum

these rays produces slight erythema which fades in 24 hours with no peeling or soreness of the skin. Greater exposure may cause slight burning, producing erythema which fades in two or three days, but which is painful and followed by slight peeling of the skin. Excessive doses of ultra-violet rays may make the skin red, sore, swollen and inflamed. The redness fades in about a week to be followed by a great deal of peeling. Extremely excessive doses can cause very painful blistering of the skin.

2. The production of melanin is stimulated by ultra-violet rays and tanning occurs which increases at each successive exposure. The amount of tanning depends on the normal colour of the skin; that is, the number of melanocytes normally present. Fair-skinned people do not tan easily and have a greater tendency to burn than people with darker skins.

3. Exposure to ultra-violet rays increases the rate of cell division in the stratum germinativum and is followed by an increased rate of shedding of scales from the stratum corneum, though the overall effect is to make the horny layer thicker.

4. Ultra-violet rays act on sterols in the epidermis to produce vitamin D.

5. Some bacteria on the skin surface are destroyed.

Dangers in the use of ultra-violet lamps

1. The rays are damaging to the eyes which must therefore be screened by suitable dark glasses to avoid inflammation.

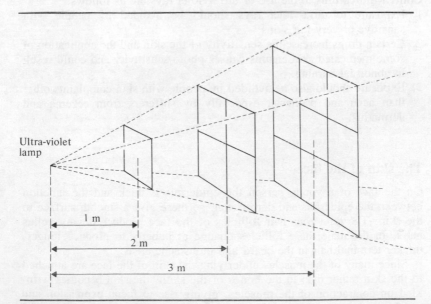

Ultra-violet lamp

1 m

2 m

3 m

Fig 2.11 The inverse square law

2. Over-exposure to ultra-violet rays can lead to burning or irritation of the skin. All areas except those requiring treatment should be covered. The manufacturer's instructions regarding time of exposure must be strictly observed.
3. Frequent exposure to ultra-violet rays both from lamps and the sun leads to premature ageing of the skin, thickening of the epidermis and increased wrinkling. Excessive exposure may lead to cancer of the skin especially of the face.
4. Some people are particularly sensitive to ultra-violet rays and react with severe itching, with dermatitis or with nausea and headaches.
5. To ensure even application of the radiation, the rays from a lamp should strike at right angles to the treatment area. For many types of lamp the intensity of radiation approximately obeys the *inverse square law*, that is the intensity of radiation varies inversely with the square of the distance from the source (see Fig. 2.11).

$$\text{Intensity of radiation (from a point source)} = \frac{1}{(\text{distance from lamp})^2}$$

The intensity at 1 metre = 4 times that at 2 metres
= 9 times that at 3 metres

Thus 4 minutes' treatment at 2 metres and 9 minutes' treatment at 3 metres will have the same effect as 1 minute at 1 metre. This law only applies when considering a point source of rays and is approximately true if the source is small.

Contra-indications to the use of ultra-violet rays are as follows:
1. Exposure to ultra-violet rays should be avoided by people with sensitive or very fair skins.
2. Certain drugs increase the sensitivity of the skin and the application of some medicated skin creams causes photo-sensitivity and could result in abnormal burning.
3. Exposure should also be avoided by people with skin complaints other than acne and psoriasis, especially by sufferers from eczema and dermatitis.

The skin of the face

On the face of a young person the epidermis is thick and the junction between the epidermis and dermis flat, so these give a smooth surface to the skin. The numerous hair follicles of the face produce downy vellus hairs. In the male these follicles change at puberty to produce longer, thicker terminal hair in the beard and moustache areas.

Since many of the muscles underlying the skin of the face are attached to the skin rather than to the bones of the skull, the skin becomes wrinkled on contraction of the muscles, giving rise to facial expression and eventually to permanent wrinkles such as frown marks, laughter lines and horizontal lines across the forehead. Excessive exposure to sunlight may also increase wrinkling as well as causing thickening of the epidermis and reduction in the elasticity of the skin leading to premature ageing.

Sebaceous glands are numerous in the face especially on the forehead and nose. They are often very large compared to vellus hair follicles and sometimes open separately from the follicles on to the surface of the skin. The large ducts of these glands are often visible particularly round the nose and may contain impacted sebaceous material, keratin scales and micro-organisms including face mites.

The skin of the face is frequently more sensitive than the skin in other areas, and allergy due to the application of para-dyes in the beard area is common in men. The skin round the eyes is often affected by allergy to nail enamel through touching the face.

The ageing of the skin

The skin of an infant is free from creases and has a soft velvety surface. Flexure lines are acquired after birth. At adolescence changes take place due to increased hormone levels. Sebaceous secretion increases, some-times leading to acne, and changes in hair growth patterns take place in the axilla and pubic regions and, in males, in the beard area.

By the mid-thirties expression lines on the face become permanent, e.g. frown lines and laughter lines. The skin gradually begins to lose its firmness since the ground substance of the dermis holds less water. The amount of fibrous tissue in the dermis increases but becomes less elastic, leading to wrinkling of the skin and the sagging of tissue. Loss of muscle tone also causes sagging of the skin and the development of a crepe effect particularly in the neck area. The natural lines of expression deepen with age.

In the fifties the epidermis becomes thinner, having fewer layers of cells, and the ridges between the epidermis and dermis become shal-lower. In females, the activity of the sebaceous glands is reduced at the menopause and the skin tends to become drier. Changes may also occur to skin colour as the number of melanocytes decreases and they become less active. Mottling of the skin sometimes results as some epidermal cells lose contact with the melanocytes. Skin tags may appear particularly on the neck, and age spots sometimes occur on the backs of the hands and on the face. In old age loss of subcutaneous fat may take place, giving less support to the skin and altering the contours of the face.

Premature ageing of the skin may be caused by over-exposure to the sun and wind, or by illness or mental stress.

Questions

1. Explain the term 'seborrhoeic areas of the skin' and give examples of these areas.

2. What is meant by the 'acid-mantle' of the skin?
3. Name:
   (a) two appendages of the skin;   (b) one area of the skin with no
   sebaceous glands;   (c) the two layers of the dermis.
4. What is the composition of sweat? Explain its main function.
5. (a) Give one possible reason why ringworm is more common in
      children than in adults.
   (b) What are the main causes of premature ageing of the skin of the
      face?
6. Describe the various effects of ultra-violet radiation on the skin.
   What precautions should be taken when using an ultra-violet lamp?
7. Explain how the skin:
   (a) acts as a protective barrier for the body;   (b) reacts if the
   salon temperature becomes abnormally high.
8. Discuss the factors which affect the colour of the skin.
9. Describe the continual changes which take place in the cells of the
   epidermis.
10. What is the function of:
   (a) the motor nerves in the skin;   (b) the sebaceous secretion;
   (c) the phagocytes in the dermis?

Chapter 3

Skin disorders

The skin normally carries a large number of bacteria and other micro-organisms on its surface, especially in folds of the skin such as the arm-pits and groin. Many of these organisms are harmless, but others are *pathogens* which could cause disease if they entered the tissues. The flaking surface of the epidermis provides a suitable breeding ground for such micro-organisms, but the thickness and compactness of the epidermis and the presence of acid secretions discourages the growth and entry of the organisms into the tissues. Some of the organisms are lost due to the constant shedding of surface scales of skin.

If the skin surface becomes broken easy entry is possible, and may lead to disease. Breakage may be caused by mechanical damage such as cuts and abrasions, or by traumas such as burns or scalds. Infestation of the skin by parasites also leads to skin breaks with consequent bacterial infection. The skin may also be irritated by contact with chemicals or by adverse weather conditions such as cold winds or excessive sun.

Some skin disorders are not caused by micro-organisms but may be due to internal or physiological abnormality such as the malfunctioning of enzyme systems which cause psoriasis.

Often a *predisposing* or contributing factor is present, making a person more susceptible to a particular disease at a particular time. For instance, damage to the skin by cuts, scratching or rubbing is a predisposing factor to the entry of bacteria into the skin and the development of boils; the increase of sebum at puberty predisposes the development of acne.

Lesions of the skin

Disorders of the skin may result in changes taking place in the surface tissues giving rise to a blemish or *lesion*. Various types of lesions are listed below and illustrated diagramatically in Fig. 3.1.

Surface of skin	Papule	Vesicle	Scales	Fissure
	Macule	Pustule	Blister	Crust

Fig 3.1 Types of lesion

A **macule** is a small abnormally coloured area of the skin, but is level with the skin surface so can be seen but not felt, e.g. a freckle.

A **papule** is a small, raised solid but unbroken part of the skin which often develops into a pustule.

A **pustule** consists of a small collection of pus which is visible through the raised epidermis. A pustule is usually accompanied by inflammation.

A **vesicle** is a small blister raised above the surface of the skin but situated in or immediately below the epidermis, and which contains a clear liquid called serum.

A **blister** is similar to, but larger than, a vesicle being raised above skin level and containing serum.

Scales consist of an accumulation of flakes of epidermis which may be imperfectly formed.

Crusts are scabs of dried serum or pus with blood, bacteria and epidermal scales. These often follow vesicles or pustules.

Fissures are cracks in the epidermis exposing the dermis.

Scars may be left after the healing of wounds has taken place.

Other effects of skin diseases include:

Erythema or areas of redness of the skin due to dilation of blood capillaries just below the epidermis.

Hyperaemia which means an increased blood flow to an area and results in erythema.

Weeping is a continuous discharge of watery liquid (serum) from an area of broken skin.

Oedema is the swelling of tissues due to an accumulation of fluid.

Inflammation of skin tissue may be accompanied by redness, swelling, pain and heat. Inflammation is due to an increase in the blood supply to an infected area of the skin. The blood vessels dilate, causing erythema and an increase in temperature in the area. The invading bacteria are attacked by white cells some of which may be killed along with bacteria, resulting in the formation of a core of pus or a 'head' through which the pus is eventually discharged. Epidermal cells (basal cells) multiply to repair the surface of the skin but a scar may result if the dermis has been damaged.

Infectious diseases

An infectious disease is one which can be passed from one person to another by the transfer of *micro-organisms*. These micro-organisms may be classified as *fungi, bacteria and viruses*. Fungi tend to grow on the outside of the body, causing such diseases as ringworm. Bacteria and viruses cause disease when they enter the body tissues and multiply there. Bacteria produce toxins which destroy body cells, whilst viruses multiply inside the cells, eventually breaking down the cell itself. These micro-organisms may enter the body through the mouth or nose thus infecting the throat, lungs or digestive tract, or through breaks in the skin leading to diseases such as impetigo. Bacteria may also multiply inside the hair follicles giving rise to boils, folliculitis and to the formation of pustules as in acne.

The body defends itself from infection by means of:

1. *Phagocytes* or wandering white blood cells which surround and digest bacteria.
2. The production of chemical *antibodies* which attack the organisms, and *antitoxins* which counteract the effect of the poisons produced by bacteria.
3. Raising body temperature which speeds up the chemical reactions required for attack on the invading organisms.

Organisms may be transmitted from person to person by the following methods:

1. **By direct contact** with an infected person:
(a) By droplet infection through inhaling air-borne droplets which are ejected from the nose or mouth of the infected person whilst coughing, sneezing or talking. Overcrowding and poor ventilation are predisposing factors to this type of infection.
(b) By touching an infected area of the body, for example whilst dressing a boil or whilst a hairdresser is attending to an infected client.
2. **By indirect contact** with an infected article such as a towel or brush. Many skin diseases are spread in this way. Infection may also be spread indirectly through infected animals such as lice, rats or mice, and via contaminated food and water.

Micro-organisms causing infection

Bacteria

Bacteria are minute single-celled organisms which, under favourable conditions, will reproduce by simple division of the cell every 20 minutes. Large numbers of bacteria inhabit the skin surface but many of these are harmless (non-pathogenic). Rafts of discarded skin carry bacteria and may transmit disease. Bacteria may be identified by microscopic examination and classified according to shape. *Cocci* are small round cells which may be arranged in bunches (staphylococci) or in long chains (streptococci); *bacilli* are rod-shaped, and *spirochaetes* have a spiral shape (see Fig. 3.2). Colonies of bacteria may also be grown or cultured on nutrient agar plates.

Some bacilli have fine hairs or *flagellae* projecting from their surfaces with which they propel themselves through liquids. Other bacilli form *spores* and develop a hard coat which enables them to survive high temperatures and dryness. They begin to reproduce again when conditions improve. For growth, bacteria require moisture, correct temperature, food and usually oxygen. Low temperatures tend to inhibit growth whilst at high temperatures (above 70 °C) bacteria are destroyed though not necessarily their spores. The optimum temperature for the growth of pathogens

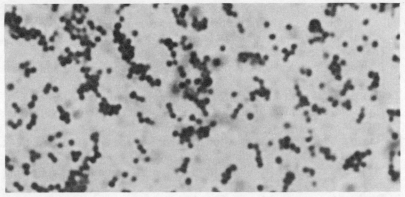

(a)

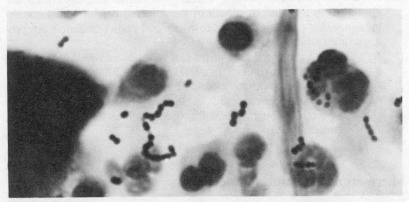

(b)

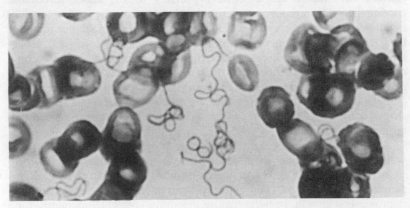

(c)

Fig 3.2 Bacteria: (a) staphylococci, (b) streptococci in pus (some bacteria being ingested by a white cell) (c) spirochaetes in blood

is about 37 °C, that is, normal body temperature. Pathogens usually favour alkaline conditions such as are found in body tissues and blood.

The bacteria affecting the skin are usually cocci which enter the tissues through cuts and other wounds.

Bacteria may be controlled in the following ways:

(a) On objects they may be destroyed by:
    (i) **chemical disinfectants**, e.g. formaldehyde in salon sterilising cabinets or cetrimide for the immersion of tools;
    (ii) **ultra-violet rays**, e.g. in salon sterilising cabinets;
    (iii) **heat** to about 70°C.

(b) On the surface of the skin they may be controlled by:
    (i) **antiseptics**, e.g. cetrimide;
    (ii) **antibiotic ointments**.

(c) Inside the body they are treated by **taking antibiotics orally or by injection** e.g. penicillin.

Viruses

Viruses are very much smaller than bacteria but can be seen by use of an electron microscope (see Fig. 3.3). In general, virus infections are more difficult to control than bacterial infections. Viruses will only multiply inside a living cell and therefore cannot be cultured on nutrient agar, in the same way as bacteria. Viruses are unaffected by antibiotics. Inside the

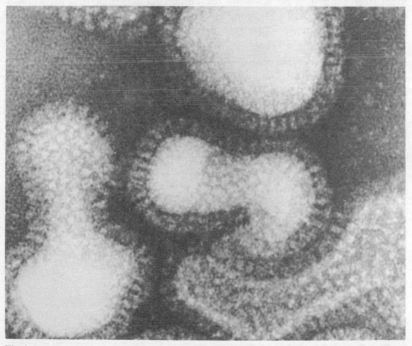

Fig 3.3 Influenza viruses

cell the viruses multiply and break down the cell, liberating the viruses to attack other cells. Since the upper layers of the epidermis are dead tissue, viruses cannot live in these areas or on the surface of the skin, but often stay for a considerable length of time in the lower epidermis, e.g. the viruses causing recurring cold sores. Viruses are destroyed in the body by antibodies which remain in the blood, usually giving subsequent immunity from the disease.

Virus infections form two main groups:

(a) Highly infectious diseases which are transmitted by direct contact through droplets of moisture or mucous from an infected person's nose or mouth, e.g. measles, influenza and common colds. The viruses survive only a short time outside body cells, and must be breathed in almost immediately if they are to infect another person.

(b) Diseases such as polio, herpes (cold sore) and warts which are not so highly infectious and where the method of transfer of infection is not so obvious. Virus infections of the skin fall in to this group.

Fungi

Fungi are a group of plants including yeasts and moulds which contain no chlorophyll in their cells and are unable therefore to make their food from water and the carbon dioxide of the air. The fungi affecting man live mostly on the surface of the skin and are parasitic. They obtain nourishment from their host by invading the epidermis and digesting the keratin of skin, nails and hair. The fungus consists of a series of fine branching threads known as a *mycelium* (see Fig. 3.4). The threads secrete a digestive juice containing a keratin-splitting enzyme.

Infection thus causes destruction of keratin which may weaken hair and nails. Irritation of the skin may result in inflammation, vesicles and pustules. The skin may also become hypersensitive to the fungus, resulting in allergic dermatitis.

Spread of fungal diseases takes place when portions of the mycelium break away and are carried directly or indirectly on to the skin of

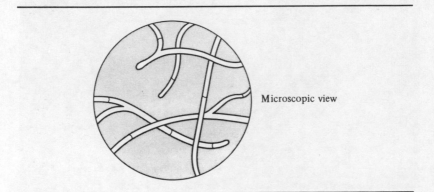

Microscopic view

Fig 3.4 The mycelium of a fungus

another person. Treatment of fungal diseases of the skin is by the drug griseofulvin, which is administered orally.

Bacterial infections of the skin

The micro-organisms responsible for bacterial infections of the skin are usually staphylococci and streptococci, both types of cocci often being present on the same site. Staphylococci cause infection deep into the skin, and are responsible for acute bacterial infection of the hair follicles called *folliculitis*, which often leads to pus formation. Infection by streptococci tends to travel along the surface of the skin, as in impetigo.

Impetigo vulgaris (or simplex)

Impetigo (see Fig. 3.5) may follow the entry of streptococci into breaks in the skin. Children are most often affected, particularly in the areas round the mouth and nose but sometimes on the scalp following infestation by lice. The infection starts with red macules which quickly form small vesicles filled with serum. These later become typical honey-coloured crusts, which are easily removed, leaving areas of moist pink skin. The infection spreads rapidly along the surface of the skin and is easily transmitted to other people by both direct and indirect contact.

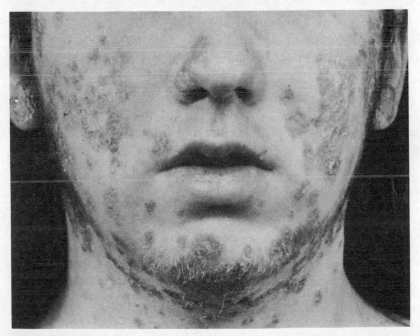

Fig 3.5 Impetigo

Staphylococcal infection may also be present leading to folliculitis and the formation of pus. Medical attention is required. Treatment usually consists of the application of antibiotic creams and the use of cetrimide shampoos. The infection usually clears in two or three weeks without leaving scars.

Brochardt's impetigo (Follicular impetigo)

Folliculitis due to staphylococcal infection of the upper part of the follicle takes the form of pustules situated at the openings of the hair follicles. Large areas of the scalp may be affected and the infection is often accompanied by enlargement of the occipital or cervical lymph nodes. The infection most frequently occurs in children and may follow infestation by lice. Treatment is by application of antibiotic ointment and the use of cetrimide shampoos.

Sycosis barbae (barber's itch)

This is a pustular folliculitis of the beard area in men and is accompanied by itching and considerable pain. It is a staphylococcal infection, often transmitted by infected razors, shaving brushes or towels. Inflammation goes deep into the dermis and the hairs in the infected area may become loose. Treatment is by antibiotic creams.

Pseudo folliculitis (ingrowing hairs)

Although this is not strictly speaking a bacterial infection it has similar characteristics. Hairs in the beard area sometimes pierce the follicle wall and cause inflammation in the dermis. The condition occurs most frequently in black skin and may be due to hair curling in the follicle, or to shaving very close, so cutting off the hair below the follicle opening enabling it to grow into the skin. The condition is known as pseudo (false) folliculitis because the inflammation is not due to infection, but to irritation of the skin by ingrowing hair. There may however be secondary infection by staphylococci and papules may be formed.

Treatment consists of epilation of the hairs by tweezers, avoidance of shaving for a time and the application of antibiotic creams to prevent secondary bacterial infection.

Furuncles (boils)

A furuncle or boil starts as a tender inflamed papule over severe folliculitis and is due to staphylococcal infection involving also inflammation of the surrounding dermis. A pustule develops and pus is later discharged from the head of the boil. Removal of the core of pus leaves a cavity which heals with a scar. Dressings and materials used to clean the site after the discharge of pus should be burned since bacteria are present.

Occasionally the inflammation subsides without the formation of a pustule and eventually disappears, the condition being known as a blind boil. Predisposing factors are poor general health, chronic complaints such as diabetes, and the rubbing of the skin especially that at the back of the neck by pressure of a collar. Boils may occur on any part of the skin including the scalp.

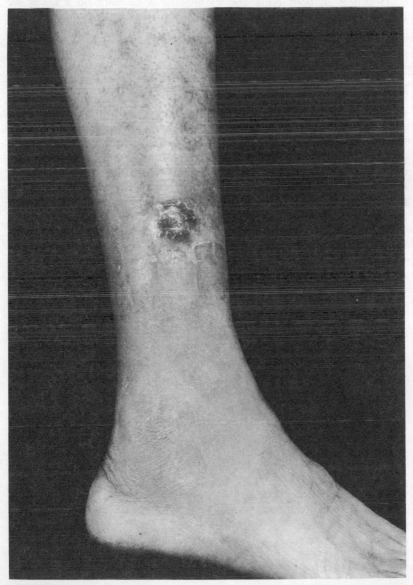

Fig 3.6 Carbuncle

Carbuncles

A carbuncle (see Fig. 3.6) is formed when several adjacent follicles are simultaneously infected by staphylococci, and is in effect a group of boils which develops several heads. Severe inflammation of the dermis also occurs.

Treatment of both boils and carbuncles is by antibiotics taken by mouth or applied locally as an ointment.

Virus infections of the skin

Herpes simplex (cold sore)

Cold sore (see Fig. 3.7) is a recurring condition due to the presence of a virus in the lower living layers of the epidermis of the lip. The infection is usually contracted in childhood, the virus remaining in the skin over a considerable period of time. The symptoms however only appear in times of stress or if the person is over-tired, has a minor illness such as a cold, or has been over-exposed to the wind or sun. It begins as an itchy red patch followed by blisters, later developing into a crust which oozes moisture.

There is no specific treatment but the condition usually clears after a few days. Care must be taken to avoid secondary bacterial infection. The complaint may be passed on from the sufferer through direct contact such as by kissing, or indirect contact through use of an infected object such as a cup or towel.

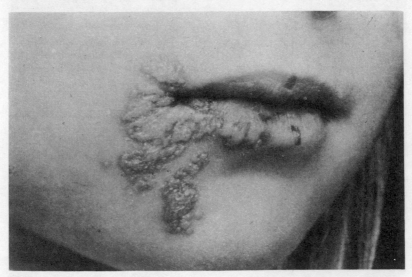

Fig 3.7 Herpes simplex (cold sore)

Herpes zoster (shingles)

The onset of shingles is marked by itching and erythema of the skin. Vesicles then develop in groups along the pathway of a sensory nerve in any part of the body. If the ophthalmic branch of the trigeminal nerve is affected, vesicles may appear on the scalp. The vesicles dry up without rupture, leaving a crust. The condition lasts for about 2 weeks but is very painful and the pain may persist. In severe cases pustules may form due to secondary bacterial infection, and scarring may occur leading to small permanently bald patches on the scalp. Shingles often occurs in adults who suffered from chicken-pox as children. Medical attention is required.

Verrucae (warts)

A virus infection in the lower living layer of the epidermis and causing a rapid increase in the number of cells in the stratum spinosum results in a small growth or wart which is raised above the surface of the skin, (except in plantar warts which grow into the skin). Abnormal keratinisation takes place, the cell nuclei are not removed and the granular layer of the epidermis is absent in the wart area. The epidermal cells of the wart also penetrate deeply into the dermis. Warts often disappear without treatment but as they are contagious they are best removed by a doctor. Solid carbon dioxide, diathermy, or electrocautery may be used for wart removal.

Plane or juvenile warts often occur in large numbers on the backs of the hands, the knees, fingers or face (mainly at the hairline), particularly

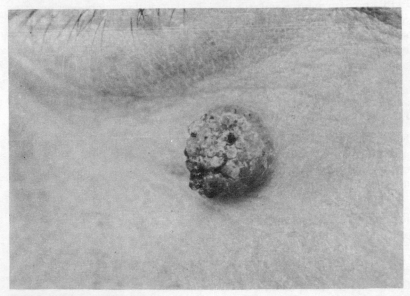

Fig 3.8 Common wart (facial)

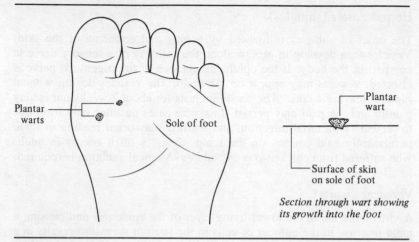

Plantar warts

Sole of foot

Plantar wart

Surface of skin on sole of foot

Section through wart showing its growth into the foot

Fig 3.9 Plantar warts

in children. The warts are raised about 1 mm above the surface of the skin, are usually round (about 5 mm in diameter) or oval in shape, flat-topped and of normal skin colour.

Common warts (Verrucae vulgaris) are usually larger than plane warts and have a much rougher surface (see Fig. 3.8). They may occur at any age but are most common in children and young adults. The most usual sites are the face or hands especially round the nails where the virus becomes implanted in hang nails.

Plantar warts grow inwards into the skin of the weight-bearing areas of the soles of the feet (see Fig. 3.9). Unlike other warts, they are usually painful due to pressure when walking. The infection is spread by people walking barefoot in public places such as beaches and swimming pools. Planter warts may be treated by a chiropodist.

Fungal infections of the skin

Fungal infections of the skin are all forms of ringworm. The fungus lives parasitically by digestion of keratin, and may therefore affect the epidermis of the skin, the hair or the nails. Ringworm of the nail is considered in Chapter 12.

Ringworm of the scalp (Tinea capitis)

Children up to the age of 12 are the most likely group to be infected by ringworm fungus. After that age the production of sebum, which is slightly fungicidal, increases and protects the skin from infection. The fungus attacks the epidermis of the scalp, enters the hair follicles and the hair shafts themselves. Enzymes produced by the fungus digest keratin,

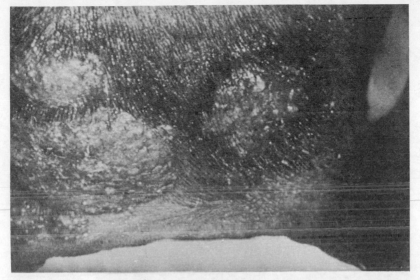

Fig 3.10 Ringworm of the scalp

causing weakening of the hair shafts, and hair breakages close to the head result in partially bald patches usually no more than 5 cm in diameter (see Fig. 3.10). Any remaining hairs on the patch appear dull and grey near the scalp due to the mycelium of the fungus.

The skin in the area becomes covered with greyish-white scales and may become inflamed, the amount of inflammation varying with the type of fungus. Animal types of ringworm, contracted from horses or domestic pets, which are mostly responsible for outbreaks of ringworm in adults, cause greater inflammation than the commoner type in children which affects only humans.

Ringworm fungus is usually passed from child to child by direct contact with an infected head, or indirectly through wearing each other's caps or by infected hairs on brushes or towels. Ringworm is rarely seen in salons, but if it is suspected no hairdressing service should be given and the client should be advised to seek medical attention.

Two other rarer types of ringworm may also affect the scalp.

Black dot ringworm causes small irregular bald patches usually less than 3 cm across and studded with black dots, which are the ends of hairs broken off slightly below skin level. Vesicles and pustules may occur leading to permanently bald patches.

Favus (honeycomb ringworm) starts as a small red macule which later develops vesicles and then characteristic sulphur-yellow concave crusts or scutula, which become embedded in the skin each surrounding a hair. A mouse-like odour is produced. The skin below the scutula becomes red and oozes moisture. Acute inflammation may occur, leading to loss of hair and some permanent bald patches.

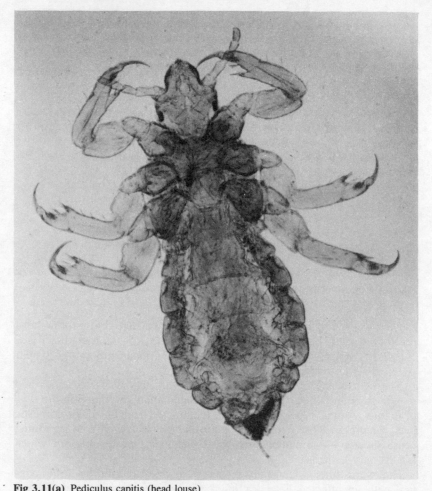

Fig 3.11(a) Pediculus capitis (head louse)

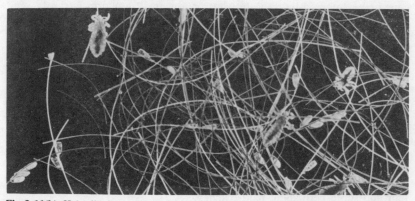

Fig 3.11(b) Hair clippings with head lice and nits

The detection of ringworm

The common type of ringworm and favus, but not black dot ringworm, may be detected by examination of the scalp under a *Wood's light*. This is an ultra-violet lamp fitted with a nickel oxide filter which allows only certain wavelengths of ultra-violet rays to pass through. The common fungus fluoresces with a greenish glow whilst favus fluoresces with a yellowish light. Fluorescence is due to the absorption of ultra-violet rays, and their conversion to rays of longer wavelength so producing visible light.

The treatment of ringworm

Ringworm is treated by an antibiotic drug, *griseofulvin*, administered orally. The drug circulates in the blood stream and is taken up by newly formed keratin of the skin, hair and nails. The new keratin is thus protected from fungal attack. By using Wood's light, the infected hair can be cut from time to time over a period of 3 months to ensure complete removal of all traces of fungus.

Ringworm of the beard (Tinea barbae)

The usual fungus causing ringworm of the beard is passed on from an animal source such as a cow or horse. The infected area becomes inflamed with the formation of papules and nodules which may grow very large, forming purplish lumps in the skin. There may be some permanent loss of hair. Treatment is by oral administration of the drug griseofulvin. Secondary infection by staphylococci may take place, the condition then being known as Tinea sycosis.

Ringworm of the body (Tinea corporis)

Red scaly circular patches occur on the trunk or limbs. These spread outwards and then heal from the centre, leaving a ring. Vesicles and pustules may occur especially if the disease has been contracted from an animal. Treatment is by oral administration of griseofulvin.

Infestation by animal parasites

A *parasite* is a living organism which lives in or on the body of a second organism, taking nourishment from the tissues of the host. Organisms living on the surface of the body are ectoparasites and those living within the host's body are endoparasites. It is the ectoparasites such as lice, fleas, itch mites and face mites that most concern the hairdresser. The presence of parasites on the human body is known as an *infestation*. This is not an infection in itself but often leads to secondary infection by bacteria, causing boils or impetigo. Bacteria may be injected into the skin when the parasite pierces the skin to obtain nourishment, or may enter breaks caused by scratching as the host attempts to relieve itching. Lice may sometimes carry typhus fever and fleas carry the plague, but these diseases are now rare.

Infestation by lice

The condition in which the body becomes infested with pediculi or lice is known as pediculosis.

There are three types of louse:

The head louse (Pediculus capitis) which infests the scalp (see Fig. 3.11).

Fig 3.12 The crab louse

The body louse (Pediculus corporis) which is similar in shape to, though slightly larger than, the head louse. This louse lives on the underclothing, laying its eggs in the clothing and taking nourishment by piercing the skin of the host and sucking blood.

The crab louse (Phthirus pubis) is smaller but slightly broader than those of the other two types, and is much rarer (see Fig. 3.12). The lice live in the pubic hairs but may occasionally be found on the eyelashes or eyebrows of children.

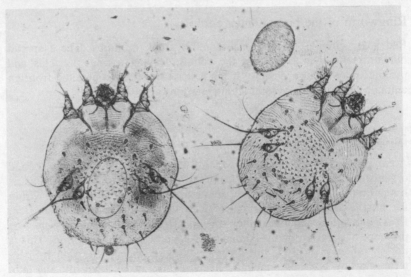

Fig 3.13 Itch mite (Sarcoptes scabiei hominis)

Pediculosis capitis

The head louse is the only type of louse of real concern to the hairdresser, and the number of cases of infestation by these parasites has increased in recent years particularly amongst children, due to the parasites acquired immunity to the insecticide DDT. DDT is now considered unsafe.

Head lice are usually found in the hair of the occipital region of the scalp but in severe cases the lice spread also to the parietal region. The adult female is about 3 mm in length and 1 mm in breadth and the male is slightly smaller. Lice have six legs each ending in a claw enabling the louse to cling easily to the hair shafts. The mouth parts of the insects are adapted for piercing the skin and sucking the blood of the host. A female louse lays about 300 eggs or *nits* in a life of about 4–5 weeks. The small shiny white oval eggs are laid close to the scalp for warmth and are firmly attached to hairs by a gummy cement secreted from the female's body. The eggs hatch in about a week, and the young take a week to mature and are then capable of reproduction. Any nits found at a greater distance than about 2 cm from the scalp are usually empty, the eggs having hatched during the time taken for the growth of the hair. Impetigo often occurs as a secondary bacterial infection in the occipital region of a scalp which is infested by lice.

Pediculosis may be treated by either applying a lotion or using a cream shampoo containing an insecticide such as *Malathion*. Several treatments are required over a period of weeks. Malathion is substantive to hair, that is it clings to keratin electrostatically and thus has a long-lasting effect. Both nits and lice are killed by the insecticide, but the nit cases are difficult to remove from the hair shafts. The cement may be softened by use of acetic acid or vinegar, and the cases detached by sliding them along the hair shaft from root to point using a fine tooth comb.

If a client is found to be infested by lice no hairdressing service should be given, as the parasites are easily transmitted to others on combs, brushes or gowns, etc. The client should be advised about treatment, and any equipment used on the client should be immediately disinfected.

Infestation by itch mites

The *itch mite* (Sarcoptes scabiei) is a small eight-legged parasite causing a condition known as *scabies* (see Fig. 3.13). The mites are just visible to the naked eye, the female being about 0.3 mm long and 0.2 mm wide, and the male slightly smaller. The female burrows into the stratum corneum of the epidermis, laying about 40–50 eggs in the burrows (see Fig. 3.15). The eggs hatch after about a week and the larvae, which are similar to the adults but have only six legs, leave the burrow to wander on the surface of the skin, and live in the hair follicles until they mature after about 6 weeks. The burrows, usually about 1 cm in length, can be seen as dark raised lines under the skin, often between the fingers, in front of the wrists, on the inside of the elbows or wherever the skin is wrinkled. Small lumps or blisters may appear over the burrows. Intense

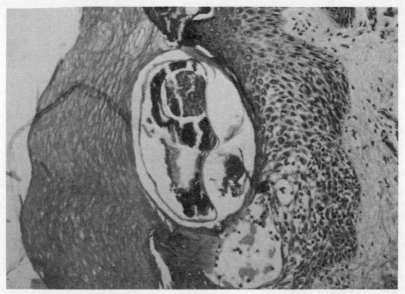

Fig 3.14 Section showing itch mite in burrow

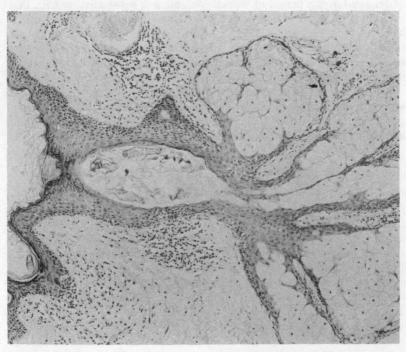

Fig 3.15 Demodex face mite in the duct of a sebaceous gland

irritation is caused, especially at night when the body is warm in bed. Impetigo or boils may result from bacterial infection of scratches. Scabies is easily transmitted from person to person by direct contact or by contact with infested objects such as sheets and blankets. Medical treatment is required. This often takes the form of application of an emulsion containing 25 per cent benzyl benzoate rubbed over the body after a hot bath. The treatment should be repeated after a few days.

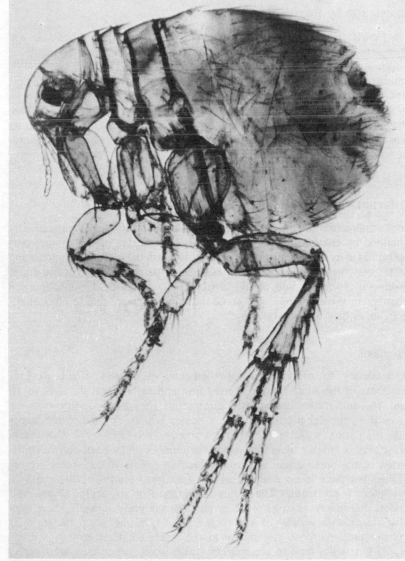

Fig 3.16 The common flea (Pulex irritans)

Infestation by face mites

The *face mite* (Demodex folliculorum), feeds on sebum and inhabits the follicles of the eyelashes and of the nose, chin and forehead, particularly if blackheads are present. The mites are about 0.3 mm in length and have four pairs of short legs and an elongated abdomen (see Fig. 3.15). As far as is known, face mites are harmless.

Infestation by fleas

The *flea* (*Pulex irritans*) is a wingless insect with a flattened body. Its six legs are well adapted for jumping and its mouthparts are adapted for biting and sucking the blood of its host (see Fig. 3.16). The bites cause small red spots surrounded by pink patches, and produce intense irritation. Breeding takes place away from the host and eggs are laid in cracks or dust, but the flea must find a host for feeding purposes. The flea moves easily from person to person by jumping, and can be eliminated by washing clothing and bedding, and cleaning rooms to remove dust, etc. in which breeding may take place.

Internal malfunctioning of the skin

In normal epidermis the cells of the basal layer multiply and are gradually changed by enzyme action to the hard keratin scales of the stratum corneum, as they travel upwards to the surface of the skin. Malfunctioning of the enzymes causes abnormalities in the type and number of the scales produced. Psoriasis and pityriasis (dandruff) are both due to abnormal changes in the epidermis, and since the conditions are due to physiological causes they are non-infectious.

Psoriasis

A tendency to psoriasis is inherited and it usually affects several members of the same family. It may first appear between the ages of 10 and 16, and recurs periodically throughout life. The condition occurs as oval or circular patches of silvery scales which are thicker and larger than the normal scales of the stratum corneum (see Fig. 3.17). The underlying skin is red due to an increase in the number and size of dermal capillaries in the area. There are small bleeding points if the scales are removed but there is no weeping of the area, no vesicles occur, and as a rule there is no itching. The scales often occur on the scalp, elbows and knees, and in severe cases on other parts of the body as well. There may also be *thimble pitting* of the finger nails. On the scalp the circular patches may encroach slightly on to the forehead. Hair growth is unaffected but scales tend to accumulate on the scalp, since they are trapped by the hair. Psoriasis is due to faulty enzyme systems in the granular

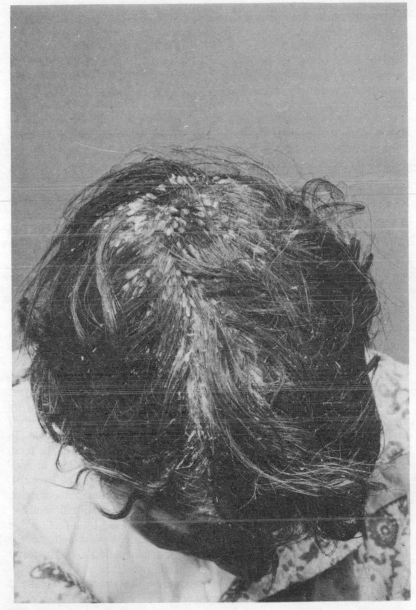

Fig 3.17 Psoriasis of the scalp

layer or to the absence of this layer, resulting in an abnormal formation of keratin. The cell nuclei are not removed and there is also an increase in the rate of cell production in the basal layer. The patches sometimes clear especially in summertime, due to the action of ultra-violet rays in sun-

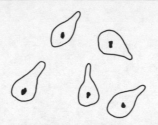

Fig 3.18 Pityrosporum ovale (bottle bacilli)

light, but they tend to recur particularly in times of stress, indicating some nervous origin of the disease. Medical advice is required. The traditional treatment was the removal of scales by use of coal tar and salicylic acid ointment. Recent treatments include irradiation with ultra-violet rays to release the enzymes of the granular layer, application of vitamin A to help to establish a granular layer and treatment with triamcinolone (a steroid) to reduce cell division. Since the condition is non-infectious, normal hairdressing services may be carried out.

Dandruff (Pityriasis simplex or sicca)

Dandruff is a non-inflammatory condition which may first appear in childhood between the ages of 6 and 10 years or at puberty. It tends to occur in people with greasy, freely perspiring skins. The condition consists of an abnormally excessive production of scales in the stratum corneum, due to an increase in the rate of cell division in the basal layer. Dry white scales may accumulate on the scalp, held to some extent by the presence of hairs. Considerable itching may be experienced. Dandruff first occurs in patches which may later join to cover the whole scalp. In severe cases the scales constantly drop to the shoulders and over the face, sometimes resulting in *blepharitis* (inflammation of the eyelids) or *conjunctivitis* (inflammation of the mucous membrane covering the eyeball). The scales are not individual cells but flakes containing hundreds of cells. In cases of dandruff the flakes tend to be larger than on normal heads.

At one time it was thought that dandruff was caused by infection due to the sharp increase in the numbers of bacteria and yeast cells on the scalp. This increase in micro-organisms is now considered to be the result of dandruff and not its cause. Excessive scaling produces an ideal breeding ground, since the sweat provides moisture, sebum the nourishment and the heat of the scalp the warmth necessary for reproduction. The population of yeast cells known as *pityrosporum ovale or 'bottle bacilli'* (see Fig. 3.18) may double in severe dandruff, and staphylococci also flourish. Dandruff tends to disappear in old age due to a lower turn-over in epidermal cells.

Cetrimide shampoos and medicated shampoos containing antiseptics such as hexachlorophane are beneficial in controlling micro-organisms

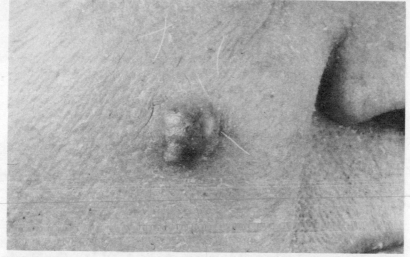

Fig 3.19 Mole

but will not cure dandruff. Modern anti-dandruff shampoos contain *selenium sulphide* or *zinc pyrithione*, which reduce cell division in the germinating layer. Frequent use of selenium sulphide can lead to dermatitis, and the substance is also damaging to the eyes. Zinc pyrithione is an antiseptic which is substantive to hair and is very effective in controlling dandruff.

Simple dandruff may be complicated by the exudation of a thin yellow serous liquid from the scalp, and the condition is then known as *pityriasis steatoides*. The scales adhere to form a waxy yellow crust. The skin may be slightly red and moist if the scales are removed. Dandruff may also be complicated by overactivity of the sebaceous glands, resulting in oily patches of scale. An aggravated form of greasy dandruff is known as *seborrhoeic dermatitis* which is considered later in this chapter as a disorder of the sebaceous glands.

Hypertrophies of the skin

Hypertrophies or excessive new growths of the skin are the result of abnormal growth of cells and usually result in small skin blemishes.

Moles (see Fig. 3.19) consist of accumulations of cells related to melanocytes which lie deep in the dermis and contain varing amounts of pigment but no blood vessels. The mole may be present at birth or may appear later by growth of cells which were already in the skin at birth. Moles are slightly raised above the surface of the skin forming flat-topped, soft swellings which may be pigmented. At puberty they often become darker and may show abnormal hair growth. If awkwardly placed, for example in the beard area, they may be surgically removed.

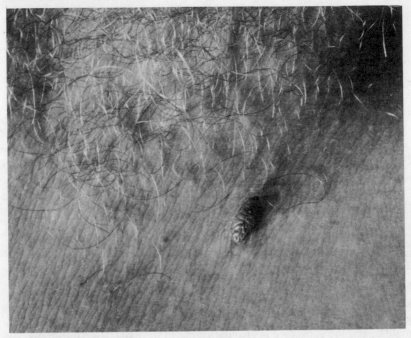

Fig 3.20 Skin tags

Otherwise they should not be interfered with as they occasionally become cancerous. If a pigmented area appears round a mole or there is any change in its size, medical advice should be sought.

Skin tags (see Fig. 3.20) often appear on the neck area and consist of small growths of fibrous tissue which stand away from the skin. They are associated with ageing and are sometimes pigmented brown or black, which makes them more obvious. They may be removed surgically if desired.

Conditions caused by external irritation of the skin

Reactions may take place in the skin to both mechanical and chemical irritation of the surface of the skin.

Neurodermatitis

Constant and often unconscious irritation of the skin by scratching may result in scaly patches, thickening of the skin and the development of waxy-looking plaques under the surface. The occipital area of the scalp is the usual site and scaling may extend from the nape of the neck to the ears, and also into the hair. The condition most frequently occurs in

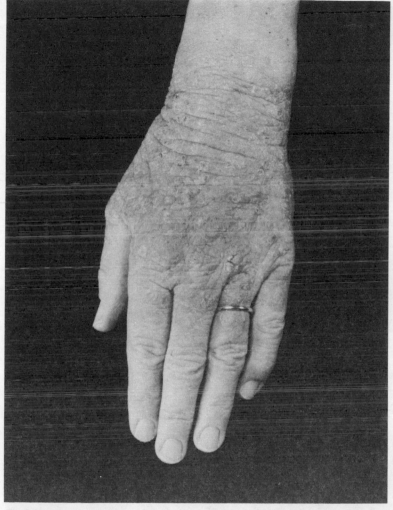

Fig 3.21 Contact dermatitis

middle-aged women and the scratching is of nervous origin. The patch clears if the irritation is discontinued.

Allergies

An *allergy* is an abnormal reaction or *hypersensitivity* of the body tissues of an individual to a substance which does not affect the majority of people. The substance causing the reaction is called an *allergen*. Some allergens may be substances taken internally as in drugs, e.g. penicillin, or foods, e.g. eggs or strawberries. They may also be inhaled, e.g.

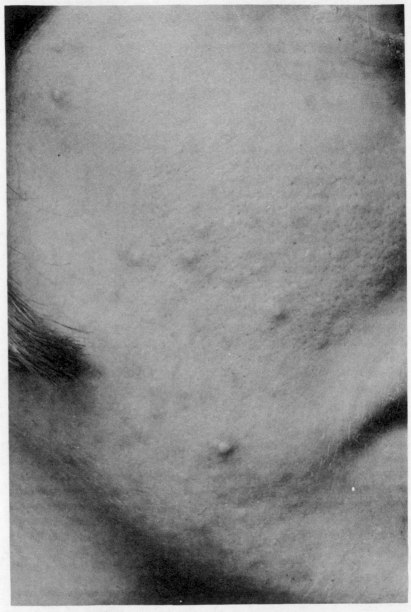

Fig 3.22 Acne vulgaris

pollen, giving rise to hay fever. Other allergens are substances which produce allergic reactions on making external contact with the skin, and it is with these substances that the hairdresser is most concerned. The external allergens give rise to *contact dermatitis* or contact eczema (see Fig. 3.21). Strictly speaking dermatitis refers to an inflammation of the skin, while eczema refers to tissue reactions involving erythema, weeping, blisters, swelling and scaling of the skin, but the two terms contact dermatitis and contact eczema are often used interchangeably.

An external chemical irritant may be a *primary irritant* if it causes inflammation of the skin at the first contact, and the irritation is limited to the area of contact. It may be a *secondary irritant* or *sensitiser* if it causes inflammation only in particular people who have become allergic to that substance through previous contact. In this case the reaction may be delayed and not confined to the area of contact. On first exposure the sensitiser produces no visible sign of irritation but causes the production of antibodies in the blood, which then react against the substance at any subsequent application. The body thus becomes allergic to that substance. The reaction to the substance may involve slight erythema or may result in the formation of vesicles with weeping and swelling of the tissues. Once the skin produces an allergic reaction to a substance, that substance or allergen should never be applied to the skin again. The hairdressing products which may cause contact dermatitis or contact eczema include: sodium lauryl sulphate (shampoo); para dyes; ammonium thioglycollate (cold wave lotion); lanolin; perfumes, especially oil of bergamot, lavender and cedarwood; formaldelyde resin (nail lacquer).

Disorders of the sweat glands

Most disorders of the sweat glands are rare, the main problem being that of excessive perspiration particularly of the feet and axillae, which may cause embarrassment due to odour and in the case of the axillae to the wetting of underarm clothing. Medical attention is required for the rarer disorders and may also be helpful in cases of abnormally excessive secretion of perspiration.

Anidrosis (lack of sweat)

Congenital lack of sweat glands occurs very rarely but leads to anidrosis or lack of perspiration. It is more often the result of some other disease such as prickly heat. The skin must be kept supple by the application of emollients.

Hyperidrosis (excessive perspiration)

Excessive perspiration is usually limited to the areas of the hands, feet and axillae where sweat glands are most numerous. It may be a congenital condition but is usually an emotional problem, since the sweat glands are under nervous control. Secretions of perspiration with a particularly offensive odour (bromidrosis) may be an added complication and is due to bacterial infection of the glands. The secretion produced by the apocrine glands of the axillae is readily attacked by the bacteria, which break it down to substances with unpleasant odours. Excessive perspiration should be treated by frequent bathing and the use of astringents such as alcohol and alum, and the liberal use of dusting powder (talc). Antiperspirants containing aluminium chlorhydrate may be used to check underarm perspiration, reducing it by up to 40 per cent. They are often formulated with deodorants in the form of antiseptics, such as hexachlorophane or cetrimide, to prevent the multiplication of the bacteria which cause odour by breakdown of sweat.

Prickly heat (miliaria rubra)

The symptoms of prickly heat are the itching of the skin, the production of small red vesicles and the inflammation of the sweat glands. The complaint may be caused by exposure to excessive heat, e.g. tropical conditions, or by the closure of the sweat ducts with keratin plugs. It may be treated by frequent bathing and the use of astringents and dusting powders.

Disorders of the sebaceous glands

Disorders involving the sebaceous glands may be due to under or over activity, or to the retention of sebum and keratin scales in the hair follicles with bacterial infection of the glands.

Asteatosis

Under activity of the sebaceous glands or asteatosis is rare and is usually associated with another disease such as hypothyroidism or with old age.

Seborrhoea

Over activity of the sebaceous glands is known as seborrhoea. In infants, excess sebum causes 'cradle cap' on the scalp. The oily scales may be removed by gentle rubbing with olive oil, then washing with a mild shampoo. At puberty over activity of the glands is associated with acne (see below). Excess sebum leads to lank, greasy hair and areas of greasy skin especially round the nose and on the forehead. Enlargement of the follicles round the sides of the nose and their blockage with dried sebum may be due to a deficiency of riboflavin (vitamin B_2) in the diet.

Seborrhoeic dermatitis

Scaliness of the scalp accompanied by excessive sebaceous secretion may be followed by an eczematised condition known as seborrhoeic dermatitis. A patch of yellowish-grey greasy scales becomes red underneath, the redness extending just beyond the area of scale and often occurring at the margin of the hair. The inflammation may spread on to the neck and particularly to the area behind the ears where fissures may occur. Patches may also arise on other seborrhoeic areas, e.g. in the folds round the nostrils and on the chest. The areas often have a festooned margin sometimes referred to as a flower-petal configuration which clears from the centre. Seborrhoeic dermatitis is a fluctuating complaint often aggravated by emotional stress. There may also be secondary bacterial infection. Seborrhoeic dermatitis predisposes to the development of contact dermatitis due to hair dyes. Shampooing should be avoided in all but simple seborrhoeic states. Treatment is by steroid creams or lotions, with an antibiotic such as vioform to combat secondary infection.

Comedones (blackheads)

When a plug of dried sebaceous material and keratin scales fills the opening of a follicle, a blackhead or comedo is formed. The head of the plug becomes blackened due to oxidation. Blackheads usually occur on the face, back or chest and may contain the face mite (Demodex foliculorum) though this is not the cause of the blackhead. Acne may follow blackheads if the blocked follicle becomes inflamed.

Acne vulgaris (simple acne)

Acne (see Fig. 3.22) is a chronic inflammatory disorder due to blockage of the hair follicles with sebum and keratin. Bacteria break down the fats in sebum forming fatty acids which seep into the tissues of the dermis surrounding the follicle, thus causing inflammation. If the plug becomes infected by bacteria, pustules and papules may occur. Since the normal flow of sebum is stopped, the contents of the follicle may be pushed deep into the dermis, forming a cyst which may later lead to permanent scars. Acne often starts at puberty due to hormonal stimulation of the sebaceous glands and usually clears by the age of 20. Any seborrhoeic area may be affected.

Acne is not generally thought to be affected by diet. Treatment is by frequent washing to degrease the area. Washing with 1 per cent cetrimide is useful as an antiseptic but it must be kept away from the eyes. Exposure to ultra-violet rays is beneficial since this increases cell division and causes mild peeling. Acne can be very disfiguring and medical aid is required if the condition does not quickly clear or if it becomes at all severe.

Sebaceous cysts (wens)

Retention of sebaceous material sometimes occurs and collects as a small sac under the skin. The size may vary from that of a pea to that of an egg. Sebaceous cysts may occur on any part of the body but are most frequent in the seborrhoic areas of the scalp, face or in the axillae. If on the scalp, the skin covering the cysts usually becomes devoid of hair. Some cysts have a small opening through which the contents can be squeezed out as a fatty substance with an unpleasant rancid smell. Sometimes the cyst has no opening and may be removed by incision under local anaesthetic. Sebaceous cysts are considered to be harmless, and unless very large and inconveniently placed are usually left alone.

Milia (white heads)

Milia are small hard pearly white spots formed from sebaceous material at the mouth of a follicle. They have no surface opening as the horny layer grows over the mouth of the follicle. White heads are harmless but often persist for some time especially round the eyes. Small milia can be removed using a sterilised needle.

Questions

1. Name the causative organism of:
   (a) tinea capitis;   (b) herpes simplex;   (c) impetigo.
2. What is meant by an ectoparasite? Give two examples of such parasites.
3. Name a substance used in the treatment of each of the following:
   (a) tinea capitis;   (b) pediculosis capitis;   (c) pityriasis sicca.
4. With what diseases or conditions are the following associated?
   (a) thimble pitting of the finger nails;   (b) dark raised lines under the skin between the fingers;   (c) waxy-looking plaques under the skin in the occipital region of the scalp.
5. State three ways in which the body defends itself against attack by bacteria.
6. Explain what is meant by a:
   (a) secondary infection;   (b) predisposition to a disease;
   (c) skin sensitiser;   (d) pathogen;
   Give examples in each case.
7. What features would distinguish:
   (a) a wart from a mole;   (b) psoriasis from pityriasis;
   (c) impetigo vulgaris from Brochardt's impetigo;   (d) a furuncle from a carbuncle?

8. Explain the differences between:
   (a) an infection and an infestation;   (b) a bacterium and a virus;   (c) a plane wart and a plantar wart.
9. Discuss the various scalp conditions which may arise as a result of excessive sebaceous secretion.
10. What are the causes and symptoms of acne vulgaris?
    Discuss the treatments used for this condition.

Chapter 4

Hair structure and growth

Hair grows by the multiplication of cells at the base of narrow pits in the skin known as *hair follicles*. As they pass along the follicles these living cells are modified in shape, become hardened by the formation of a tough protein called keratin, and suffer the loss of their nuclei by enzyme action leading to the death of the cell. Thus the hair shaft leaving the follicle is a dead structure composed of keratin and this is arranged in three distinct cylindrical layers. The outer layer or *cuticle* consists of overlapping scales, next is the *cortex* of spindle-shaped cells which lie parallel to the length of the hair, and in the centre is the *medulla* which consists of a honeycomb of irregularly shaped areas of keratin with air spaces between them. Granules of the pigment *melanin* situated mainly in the cortex give colour to the hair.

The angle of inclination of the follicle in the skin (see Fig. 4.1), together with the degree of stiffness of the hair, determines the hairs'

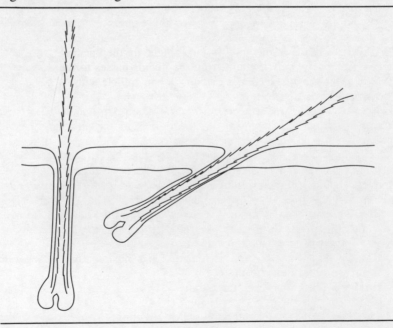

Fig 4.1 Effect of angle of inclination of hair follicle

natural lift, that is whether it tends to stand erect or lie flat on the scalp. The inclination also determines the direction of growth of the hair. The follicles of the eyelashes are at right angles to the skin surface therefore the lashes grow straight out from the skin. The eyebrows on the other hand grow from follicles which are only very slightly inclined so the eyebrows lie close to the skin and they all lie in one direction.

Scalp hairs tend to grow in groups, causing different sections of the hair to lie in different directions. At the crown for example the inclination of the follicles causes all the hairs to grow away from one point. If a natural parting exists, the hair falls easily to each side. At the front margin the hair may have a natural tendency to grow forwards, backwards or to one side. The hairdresser must consider the natural lie of the hair when planning a suitable style for a client. The lie of the hair is also important when transplants of hair are being made on bald heads.

The structure of a mature hair follicle

The follicle of a scalp hair (see Fig. 4.2) is about 4 mm deep and 0.4 mm wide. Its walls or *outer root sheath* are a continuation of the epidermis of the skin and consist of two to four rows of cells, the thickness being greater in large follicles. The lower portion of the follicle widens out into the *hair bulb* which contains the *germinal matrix*. Dermal tissue projects upwards into the base of the follicle to form the *dermal papilla* enclosing a capillary network. Amongst the cells surrounding the upper part of the papilla are *melanocytes* which produce melanin granules and distribute them into the cortical cells of the growing hair.

About two-thirds of the way up the follicle are the openings of one or more *sebaceous glands*. Sebum from the glands passes to the surface of the skin along the *pilo-sebaceous canal*. A hair follicle with its associated sebaceous glands is known as a *pilo-sebaceous unit*.

The hair muscle or *arrector pili muscle* extends from the outer root sheath about one third the way up the follicle to the underside of the epidermis. In cold conditions or in times of fear, the muscle contracts, moving the sloping follicle to make the hair stand erect. This action also causes the skin near the opening of the follicle to be raised in a 'goose pimple'. The hairs of the eyelashes and eyebrows have no erector muscles. The part of the follicle below the muscle is the temporary part of the follicle, and degenerates during the growth cycle of the hair.

Whilst in the follicle, the hair itself is surrounded and protected by an **inner root sheath** consisting of three layers:

1. **Henle's layer** of one cell in thickness lies next to, but is separate from, the outer root sheath.
2. **Huxley's layer** of two or three cells thickness is the middle layer of the sheath.
3. **The cuticle**, with overlapping scales pointing to the base of the follicle, interlocks with the cuticle of the hair.

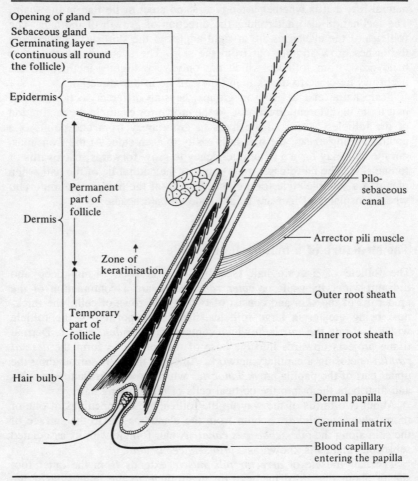

Fig 4.2 A mature hair follicle

The inner root sheath and the hair grow at the same rate and move along the follicle together. The inner root sheath breaks down at about the level of the opening of the sebaceous glands. The passage of the hair along the pilo-sebaceous canal is eased by the presence of sebum.

The development of hair follicles in the foetus

Hair follicles begin to develop in the foetus at between 8 to 12 weeks after conception. Those of the face appear first, followed by the follicles of the forehead and scalp. The follicles of the trunk and limbs appear at about 18 weeks. New follicles form amongst those first developed and

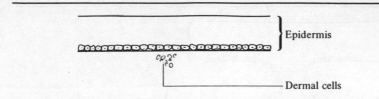

Fig 4.3 First stage in the development of a follicle

often two secondary follicles are formed near the original one to make a group of three.

Development of a follicle starts by the crowding together of a group of dermal cells just below the surface of the epidermis (see Fig. 4.3). This group of cells eventually forms the dermal papilla. By cell division in the stratum germinativum, a peg of cells is formed which pushes down the cluster of dermal cells below it. The peg grows at an angle to the surface of the skin, the outer cells of the peg being arranged neatly along the sides of the peg as a continuation of the stratum germinativum (see Fig. 4.4).

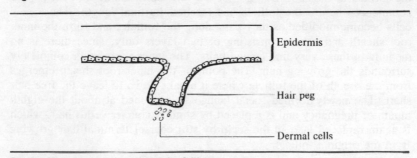

Fig 4.4 Hair peg (development of the follicle)

The lower part of the peg later broadens out to form the hair bulb, the base becoming first flattened and later slightly concave due to the pressure of the dermal cells which hollow out the base of the follicle to form the papilla. The whole follicle is made of epidermal tissue which dips down into the dermis and there is no break in the epidermis during the formation of the follicle.

Two swellings appear on the same side of the developing follicle (see Fig. 4.5). A round knob of cells pushes out from the side of the upper follicle to eventually become the sebaceous gland. A bulge or thickening of the outer coat of the peg below the round knob makes a point of attachment for the arrector pili muscle which later develops from dermal tissue.

Melanocytes are carried down from the stratum germinativium along with the peg and are finally distributed amongst the cells surrounding the upper part of the papilla. Blood capillaries gather at the lower end of the follicle and eventually enter the papilla.

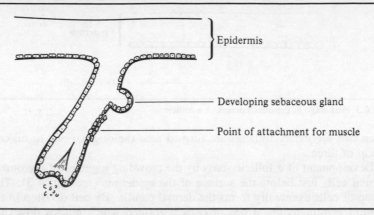

Epidermis

Developing sebaceous gland

Point of attachment for muscle

Fig 4.5 Bulge stage (development of hair follicle)

A solid core of elongated cells extends upwards through the peg to form the pilary canal through which the new hair will penetrate to reach the surface of the skin. Division of the cells surrounding the hair papilla commences before the follicle has reached its final length. These new cells become modified as they pass along the follicle, and form the inner root sheath and a hair consisting of two layers only, since there is no medulla in these very fine lanugo hairs. The inner root sheath completely surrounds the growing hair. The point of the inner root sheath emerges from the mouth of the follicle where it breaks down to leave the free hair shaft. The newly formed foetal lanugo hair is shed at about the eighth month of pregnancy and is replaced by slightly coarser vellus hair, which is again replaced later in the scalp by still coarser terminal hair growing from the original follicle.

The distribution of hair follicles in the skin

The number of follicles in the skin is fixed at birth and new follicles do not develop later. The follicles become more widely spread as the surface area increases during growth of the body. Some areas of the skin have no follicles. The *areas of glabrous skin* include the palms of the hands, soles of the feet, the lips and the terminal joints of the fingers and toes. Other areas may contain up to about 1000 follicles per square centimetre, the greatest density of hair being on the scalp and facial areas.

Follicles may be single but are often found in groups of three. In the beard areas 1 coarse terminal hair is often surrounded by several vellus type follicles.

Growth of the hair with its inner root sheath

The growth of the hair and inner root sheath takes place by the multiplication of cells in the germinal matrix which surrounds the hair papilla in the lower part of the hair bulb. As new cells are formed they push the older cells upwards. In the lower bulb all the cells are alike, but as they reach the upper bulb they become larger and begin to change shape or differentiate, to form the cells of the 3 layers of the hair and the 3 layers of the inner root sheath.

Above the bulb the follicle narrows and the developing cells are funnelled into the *zone of keratinisation*. Enzymes destroy the cell nuclei and cause the hardening of the cells by the formation of the horny protein material, keratin. By the time they are one third of the way up the follicle the cells have taken on a new shape, are dead and fully keratinised.

The development of the inner root sheath

The first cells to harden are those of Henle's layer of the inner root sheath. This is important because Henle's layer ensures the easy passage of the developing hair along the pilary canal. Henle's layer consists of a single layer of slightly elongated cells forming a smooth surface, which can readily slip over the stationary cells of the outer root sheath. The cells of Huxley's layer develop a softer type of keratin. The cuticle of the inner root sheath develops from a single row of cells from the matrix which harden at the same time as those of the hair cuticle.

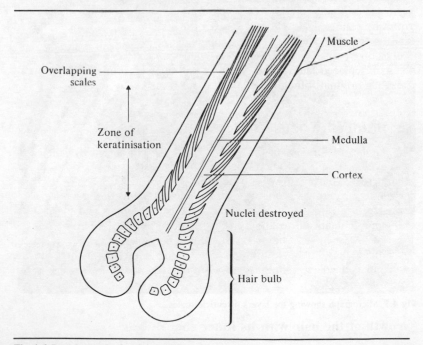

Fig 4.6 Development of cuticle scales

Development of the cuticle

A single row of cells from the germinal matrix differentiates to form the hair cuticle. In the mid-bulb these cells are roughly in the form of cubes. By the time they reach the upper bulb they are columnar (see Fig. 4.6), the longer edges pointing towards the sides of the follicle. The outer edges of the cells then become tipped upwards into a point in a direction away from the base of the follicle. The cells become longer and thinner, the nuclei disappear and the cells begin to overlap.

About halfway up the follicle they have achieved their final shape and have been hardened by the formation of keratin in the cells. Seven to eleven cells overlap each other and the points of these cells interlock with the cuticle scales of the inner root sheath (see Fig. 4.7).

The keratin in the cuticle scales consists of a twisted mass of polypeptide chains which are very rich in the amino acid cystine. The cells are free from pigment and are translucent. The edges of the scales are rounded and they lie compactly together. Cuticle cells adhere to those of the cortex and tend to hold the hair together. If the cuticle is destroyed the hair becomes easily frayed and damaged. The cuticle is said to be coronal if one scale completely surrounds the hair to form a ring, and imbricated if the scales only extend part way round the hair.

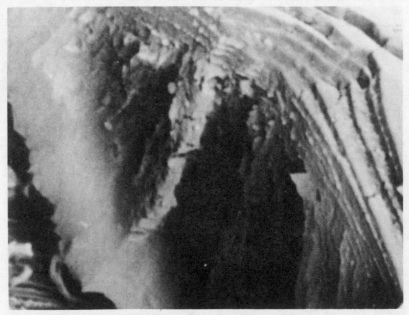

Fig 4.7 Micrograph showing the layers of cuticle scales

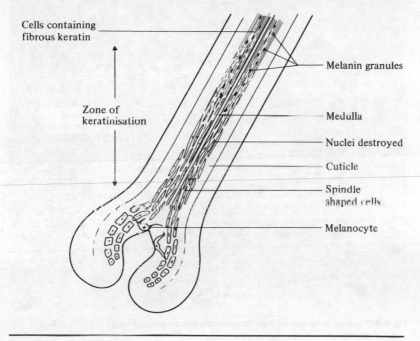

Cells containing fibrous keratin

Zone of keratinisation

Melanin granules

Medulla

Nuclei destroyed

Cuticle

Spindle shaped cells

Melanocyte

Fig 4.8 Development of the cortex

Development of the cortex

The cortex forms the main bulk of the hair and lies between the medulla in the centre of the hair and the outer cuticle. The cells which develop into the hair cortex arise from the germinal matrix in the shape of cubes. In the upper bulb they become larger and more elongated (see Fig. 4.8). Here they receive granules of the pigment melanin which are passed into the cortical cells by intercellar bridges from melanocytes in the cells surrounding the upper part of the papilla. The cortical layer is thus responsible for hair colour (see Fig. 4.9).

As the cells are funnelled from the bulb into the narrower part of the follicle they become more spindle shaped, and by the time they reach the zone of keratinisation they are long and thin. The cell nuclei are destroyed and the cells are hardened by the formation of keratin. The polypeptide chains in this type of keratin form long coils which lie parallel to the sides of the elongated cells. The cells also become fused with adjacent cells, and the polypeptide chains link up with those of adjoining cells to form long fibrils. A cystine-rich *intercellular cement* or *matrix* of twisted polypeptide chains is formed between the fibrils. The detailed chemical structure of this type of keratin is considered later in this chapter.

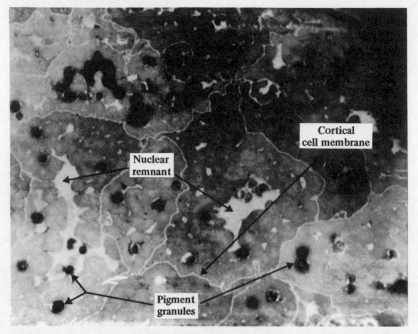

Fig 4.9 Transverse section of hair demonstrating the arrangement of cortical cells and pigmentation

Development of the medulla

The cells forming the medulla or central core of the hair develop as cuboid cells in the germinal matrix. The cells become much enlarged and since keratinisation in these cells takes place only against the cell walls, a cavity remains where the nucleus and most of the cytoplasm have broken down. This gives a fairly rigid structure to the medulla, tending to make the hair stiff (see Fig. 4.10). The medulla may be continuous or fragmented, and in very fine hair is often absent so leading to the softness of these hairs. The cells of the medulla contain little or no colour. Air spaces occur between the cells as well as within the cells themselves.

The growth cycle of hair.

Active growth of hair is not continuous throughout the life of a follicle since the follicle undergoes alternate periods of activity and periods of rest (see Fig. 4.11). In animals, many follicles enter the resting stage at the same time and the animal moults. In man, individual follicles enter the resting stage at different times so that the replacement of hair takes place gradually and there is a constant daily loss of about a hundred scalp hairs. The length of the period of active growth (anagen), the period of

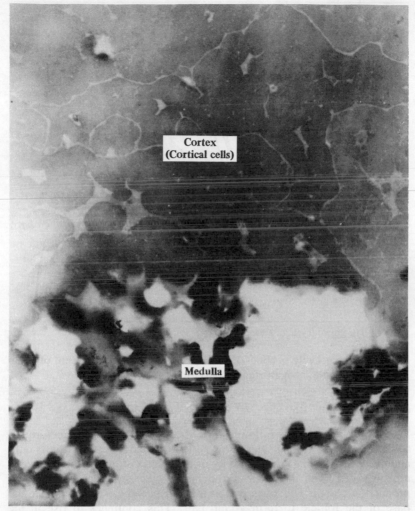

Fig 4.10 Transverse section of hair showing part of the cortex and medulla

change to the resting stage (catagen) and the resting stage itself (telogen) are all determined genetically but may be affected by hormonal changes or drugs.

Anagen

The period of active growth of scalp hairs is from 2 to 7 years. New hairs growing early in anagen grow faster than older hairs, the average rate of growth being 1.25 cm a month. Thus the maximum length of a hair undergoing a 2-year cycle is about 30 cm whilst the maximum length of a

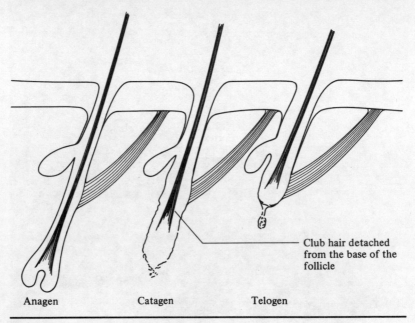

Club hair detached
from the base of the
follicle

Anagen   Catagen   Telogen

Fig 4.11 The growth cycle of a hair

hair in a 7-year cycle is about 1 metre. Eighty to ninety per cent of scalp follicles are in the anagen stage at any one time.

Catagen

The period of growth is followed by a short period of change before the follicle enters the resting stage. This period of change (catagen) lasts only about 2 weeks during which activity of the matrix stops and no new cells are produced. The dendrites of the melanocytes contract and melanin production ceases. The lower part of the hair becomes separated from the base of the follicle to form a club hair. This continues to rise in the follicle since it is attached to the inner root sheath. The lower part of the outer root sheath collapses, forming a cord or root germ attached to cells previously in the dermal papilla. The follicle becomes shorter by about one third. At any one time only about 1 per cent of scalp follicles are in catagen.

Telogen

The resting stage of the follicle, telogen, lasts 3 to 4 months. The follicle remains quiescent in its shortened state, but is still in contact with the dermal papilla through the root germ. About 13 per cent of follicles are in telogen at any one time. When the resting stage is completed, growth of the new follicle begins from the root germ. The hair bulb is reformed and a new hair starts to grow from the matrix. If the old club hair is still in the follicle it is usually pushed out by the newly growing hair as the period of anagen recommences.

The blood supply to a follicle

In a mature and active follicle a series of parallel blood vessels run along the length of the follicle. Other vessels branch from these to make networks of capillaries round the lower third of the follicle including the bulb and the zone of keratinisation. At the level of the sebaceous gland another network surrounds both the follicle and all the lobes of the gland. The vessels of the upper follicle are extensions of the papillary network in the upper dermis whilst the supply to the lower follicle is derived from larger vessels in the dermal plexus. The 2 sets of vessels join and form a network round the follicle. Some of the vertical vessels enter the hair papilla and form a loop of capillaries to bring nourishment to the growing hair (see Fig. 4.12).

The smaller the follicle the less elaborate is the blood supply. Vellus

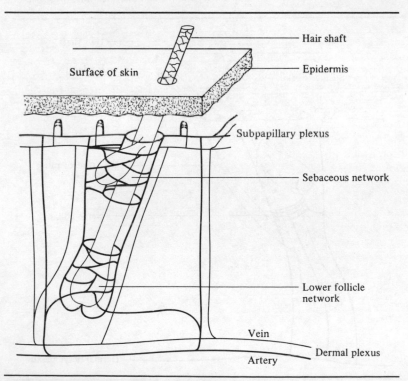

Fig 4.12 Blood supply to a follicle

hairs have few blood vessels, and none in the hair papilla. If the vellus hair has a large sebaceous gland as on some bald heads, the sebaceous gland is supplied with a dense network of capillaries.

In catagen the follicle becomes shorter and the lower part of the follicle withdraws from the surrounding capillary network. Some of the capillaries disappear, but others remain collapsed near the follicle as a tangled bundle. The vessels in the upper part of the follicle remain unchanged. When the follicle becomes active again and increases in length, the capillary networks are redeveloped.

The nerve supply to a hair follicle

Only the permanent part of the follicle has a nerve supply. This consists of a collar of sensory nerve fibres which circles the follicle just below the level of the sebaceous glands. Nerve fibres in the outer dermal coat run a straight course up the sides of the follicle to the collar, from a nerve plexus deep in the dermis (see Fig. 4.13). Branches of the collar enter the walls of the follicle making the hair sensitive to touch.

From the collar other fibres extend up to the pilo-sebaceous canal and

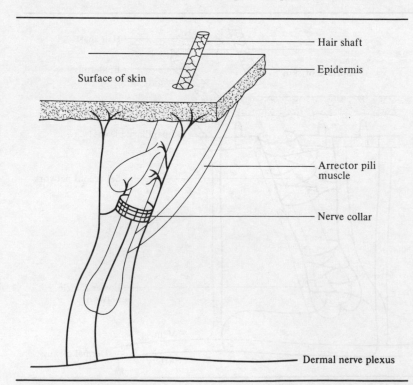

Fig 4.13 Nerve supply to a follicle

divide into fine fibres in the lower part of the epidermis. A few very fine fibres pass from the collar to the sebaceous glands and others extend to the sweat glands and the arrector pili muscles.

During telogen the collar remains intact and so the permanent part of the follicle retains its nerve supply. The follicle may partially slip out of the collar which shrinks but is still intact. In bald skin the collar may become detached from the shrunken follicle and then forms a structure similar to a Meissner's touch corpuscle.

Keratinisation and the structure of keratin

Keratin is a protein and contains the elements carbon, hydrogen, oxygen, nitrogen and sulphur. In comparison with other proteins, the sulphur content of keratin is abnormally high. Like all proteins, keratin is made up of *amino acid units* which are chemically bound together by *peptide linkages* to form long chains known as *polypeptide chains*. Amino acids are brought by tissue fluid to the developing hair cells from the blood in the capillaries of the hair papilla, and originate in the protein-containing foods of the diet. Keratinisation takes place in the area of the follicle above the bulb. Eighteen different amino acids are required to produce keratin.

All amino acids are made up of at least one amino group (a basic or 'alkali' group) and one carboxyl group (an acid group). Some amino acids, including the simplest one known as glycine, have only one amino group and one acid group. Others may have one amino group and two acid groups, or two amino groups and one acid group, or two acid and two amino groups. Representing the amino (basic) group by □ and the acid group by ■, the various types of amino acids are shown in Table 4.1.

During keratinisation, enzymes in the cells cause the amino acids to

Table 4.1 Amino acids

Types of amino acid	Example	Symbol		
One amino (basic) group and one acid group	glycine	basic group	□—■	acid group
Two amino (basic) groups and one acid group	arginine	basic group	□—■ / □ / basic group	acid group
One amino (basic) group and two acid groups	glutamic acid	basic group	□—■ / ■ / acid group	acid group
Two amino (basic) groups and two acid groups (with two sulphur atoms between the groups)	cystine	basic group acid group	□ ■ / -SS- / ■ □	acid group basic group

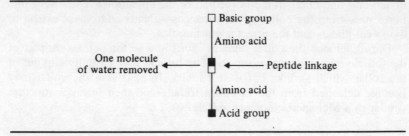

Fig 4.14 Formation of a dipeptide

join together chemically. The amino (basic) group of one amino acid joins the acidic group of a second amino acid, a molecule of water being split off between the 2 amino acids which are then joined by a peptide linkage.

Two amino acids chemically united together form *a dipeptide* (see Fig. 4.14) which also has a basic group at one end of its molecule and an acid group at the other, to which further amino acids may join. In this

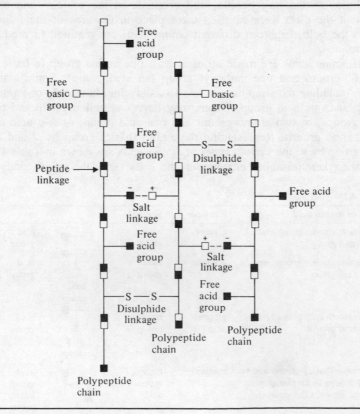

Fig 4.15 Formation of polypeptide chains

way long chains of amino acids may be built up to form a polypeptide chain (see Fig. 4.15).

In keratin, the polypeptide chains are arranged as an *alpha-helix* (α-helix) like a coiled spring, with about three or four amino acid units in each turn of the helix (see Fig. 4.16).

In the zone of keratinisation, the polypeptide chains become connected by various types of cross-linkages. These form between the coils of the chains as well as between adjacent chains.

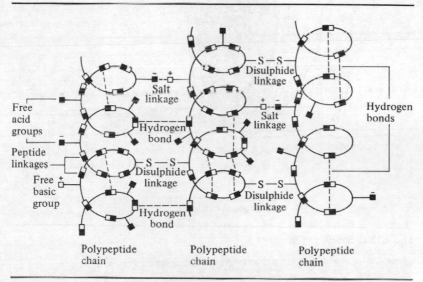

Fig 4.16 The chemical structure of keratin

Disulphide linkages

Since the amino acid cystine contains two amino groups and two acid groups, this amino acid can take part in two separate polypeptide chains forming a bridge between the two chains linked through two sulphur atoms (see Fig. 4.15). This bridge is therefore called a *disulphide linkage* or a *cystine linkage*. These linkages give keratin a ladder-like structure. The disulphide linkages are very strong and play a main part in the chemical reactions which take place during perming and hair straightening.

Salt linkages

If a free acid group (from an amino acid containing two acid groups) in 1 chain lies opposite to a free amino (basic) group in the adjacent chain the two will form a salt linkage. The two groups have opposite electrical charges and therefore are attracted to each other. This ionic or electrostatic linkage is weaker than a disulphide linkage and is easily broken by either weak acids or weak alkalis.

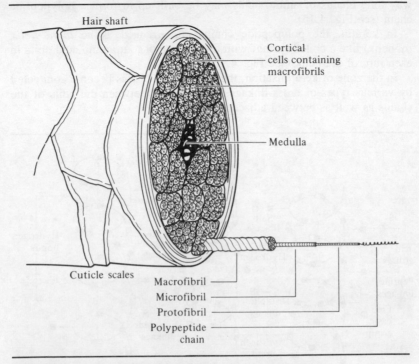

Hair shaft

Cortical
cells containing
macrofibrils

Medulla

Cuticle scales

Macrofibril

Microfibril

Protofibril

Polypeptide
chain

Fig. 4.17(a) Structure of the cortex

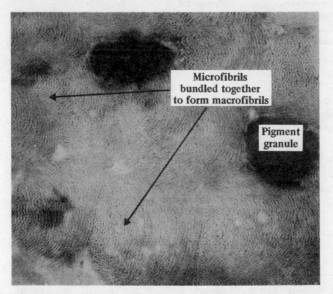

Microfibrils
bundled together
to form macrofibrils

Pigment
granule

Fig 4.17(b) Transverse section of hair showing arrangement of
macrofibrils and microfibrils

Hydrogen bonds

The coils of the polypeptide chains are held together by numerous weak hydrogen bonds, which form due to a force of attraction between a hydrogen atom in one turn of the coil and an oxygen atom lying close by in an adjacent turn. They also form between hydrogen and oxygen atoms in adjacent polypeptide chains. These bonds are important because they affect the elasticity of hair. Water molecules are able to join in the hydrogen bonds and are then known as *'bound water'*.

The structure of the cortex

In the cortex the helical polypeptide chains lie parallel to the length of the hair. Several polypeptide chains are twisted together to form a *protofibril* and several protofibrils are similarly twisted to make a *microfibril*. Bundles of microfibrils form one *macrofibril*, the largest of the *cortical fibres*. The cortical cells thus contain a series of fibres enclosing even finer fibrils, the smallest units being the polypeptic chains (see Fig. 4.17). The

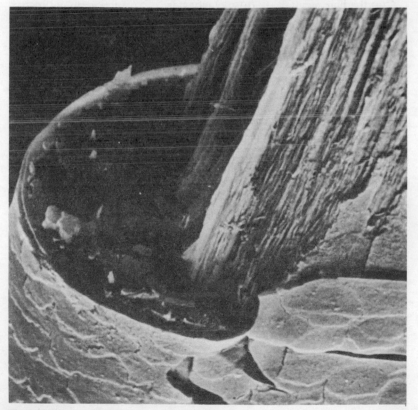

Fig 4.18 Micrograph of hair showing cuticle scales and cortical fibres

fibrils branch and join adjacent bundles of fibres to give greater strength. The cortex thus has a well organised system of parallel fibres, unlike the keratin of the cuticle in which the polypeptide chains form a twisted unorganised mass. The cortical fibres are however held together by a *matrix of intercellular cement* which is also a mass of twisted chains and very rich in cystine (see Fig. 4.18).

Questions

1. Explain the difference between:
   (a) lanugo hair and vellus hair;   (b) anagen and telogen.
2. What is meant by:
   (a) the pilary canal?   (b) intercellular bridges?   (c) intercellular cement?
3. Explain the chemical structure of:
   (a) hydrogen bonds;   (b) cystine linkages;   (c) salt linkages.
4. State the function of:
   (a) the hair papilla;   (b) melanocytes;   (c) the germinal matrix of the follicle.
5. Explain how newly formed hair is protected as it travels through the follicle.
6. Describe with the aid of diagrams the structure of the cuticle of a hair. Explain the series of changes which take place in the cells of the germinal matrix to form this structure.
7. By considering the structure of hair, explain:
   (a) what happens to the cuticle scales when a hair is stretched;   (b) why hair is hygroscopic;   (c) the factors which affect the porosity of hair.
8. Describe the structure of the inner root sheath and discuss its main functions.
9. Explain what happens to cells in:
   (a) the germinal matrix of a follicle;   (b) the upper bulb;
   (c) the zone of keratinisation.
10. By considering the chemical structure of hair explain why:
    (a) hair is elastic;   (b) hair tends to split more easily lengthways than across the hair shaft.

Chapter 5

Factors affecting hair growth

The main requirements of the cells which develop from the germinal matrix in the bulb to produce hair are as follows:

Amino acids are required for cell development and growth and also for keratinisation. These amino acids are obtained by the digestion of protein-based foods such as meat, fish, eggs, cheese and milk. Digestive enzymes, which attack the polypeptide linkages, split the proteins into individual amino acids. These are absorbed from the small intestine and circulated in the blood. The amino acids reaching the hair papillae are transferred to the developing cells by tissue fluid. Eighteen different amino acids are required to build keratin and these must all be present in the cells at the same time.

Energy is required to enable various chemical reactions to take place inside the cells. This energy is obtained during tissue respiration (internal respiration) by the *oxidation of glucose*.

$$\text{glucose} + \text{oxygen} = \text{carbon dioxide} + \text{water} + \text{energy}$$

Glucose is a type of sugar obtained mainly by the digestion of carbohydrate foods (starches and sugars) but may also be obtained by the breakdown of fats or from any amino acids not required for building new tissue. *Oxygen* enters the blood in the capillaries of the lungs during external respiration and is transported to the papillae as oxy-haemoglobin in red blood cells. Vitamins of the B group are necessary as catalysts to enable oxidation to take place at body temperature. Many other vitamins and minerals also play a part in hair growth. The passage of these substances to the hair papillae is shown in Fig. 5.1.

The growth of hair thus depends on:
(a) an adequate diet and efficient digestive system;
(b) an adequate supply of oxygen and the efficiency of the respiratory system;
(c) the circulation of the blood and transfer of nutrients and oxygen to the growing cells and the removal of waste from the cells.

Any changes in these factors, as well as alterations to the rate of cell division, e.g. by antimitotic drugs or ultra-violet radiation, and to the normal growth cycle of the follicle, will affect hair growth.

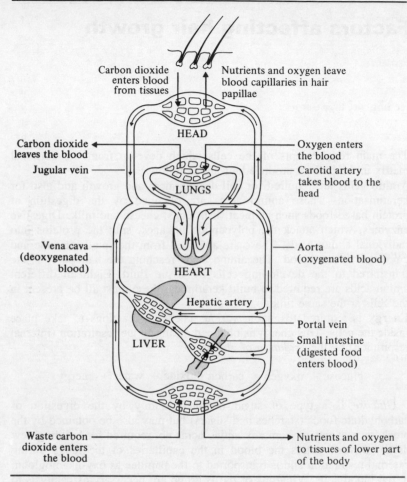

Carbon dioxide enters blood from tissues

Nutrients and oxygen leave blood capillaries in hair papillae

HEAD

Carbon dioxide leaves the blood

Jugular vein

Oxygen enters the blood

Carotid artery takes blood to the head

LUNGS

Vena cava (deoxygenated blood)

Aorta (oxygenated blood)

HEART

Hepatic artery

Portal vein

Small intestine (digested food enters blood)

LIVER

Waste carbon dioxide enters the blood

Nutrients and oxygen to tissues of lower part of the body

Fig 5.1 Distribution of nutrients and oxygen to the hair follicles

The effect of diet on hair growth

Diet can only affect the growth of newly developing hair in the follicle. The hairshaft itself is dead tissue so receives no nourishment though its condition may be affected by externally applied materials. The effect of an adequate diet is dependent on the efficiency of the digestive system, the respiratory system and the circulation of the blood as previously outlined.

Carbohydrates and fats
Carbohydrates and fats supply the body with energy but lack of these nutrients is unlikely except in conditions of extreme privation. Some

slimming diets based on high protein consumption may partially exclude carbohydrates and fats, but in that case proteins or the bodily store of fat are used to provide energy.

Protein
The effect of shortage of dietary protein is seen in children in some developing countries where infants are weaned straight from breast-feeding on to a largely carbohydrate dict. This leads to the condition known as *kwashiorkor*. The first sign of protein deficiency is loss of hair colour. Melanin is formed by the oxidation of the amino acid tyrosine, and if this is lacking in the diet melanin production is affected. Hair which is normally black becomes red due to changes in the type and amount of melanin produced. The hair may eventually lose all colour, and become thin and easily broken due to inadequate keratin formation. The diameter of the hair may be reduced by half and there may be diffuse hair loss. Lack of protein in the diet is rare in more highly developed countries.

Mineral elements
Although traces of many mineral elements are required for the correct functioning of the body, hair growth is most likely to be affected by lack of iron, calcium or iodine.

Iron is required for the formation of haemoglobin (a compound of protein and iron) in the red blood cells. Deficiency of iron in the diet causes a reduction in the number of red cells or a lowering of their haemoglobin content, and leads to anaemia. Since haemoglobin carries oxygen in the red cells the amount of oxygen reaching the hair papillae may be reduced, affecting cell division and resulting in poor hair growth.

Low levels of *calcium* in the blood lead to chronic disorders of the epidermis and the abnormal formation of keratin. This may be due to faulty diet but is more usually the result of the malfunctioning of the parathyroid gland which controls the level of calcium in the blood.

The element *iodine* is necessary for the production of the hormone thyroxine, the secretion of the thyroid gland. Shortage of iodine leads to the enlargement of the gland or goitre, but this is now rare due to the introduction of iodised table salt. A decrease of thyroxine secretion results in the slowing down of the whole working rate of body processes. Poor, thin hair is produced with some loss in the frontal regions.

Vitamins
Hair growth is affected by vitamin A, vitamin C and possibly the vitamins of the B group.

Vitamin A (retinol) is necessary for normal keratin formation and deficiency causes keratin to form on the mucous membranes of the nose, throat and the cornea of the eye, and also to accumulate at the openings of the hair follicles. The hair itself becomes dry and lustreless with possibly some diffuse hair loss. Excess of Vitamin A in the diet results in small bald patches on the scalp.

The *vitamins of the B group* are catalysts for the oxidation of glucose to produce energy for cell reactions. They have been found to affect the colour and growth of hair in animals but there is no evidence of a similar effect in man.

The presence of *vitamin C* (ascorbic acid) increases the absorption of iron from the small intestine, thus helping to prevent anaemia. It is also responsible for the formation of strong cementing material between body cells. Deficiency of vitamin C in the diet results in haemorrhages round the hair follicles which then produce abnormal keratin and often develop cork-screw hairs.

The effect of illness on hair growth

Illness can cause thinning of the hair shaft, loss of hair colour or hair-fall due to changes in the growth cycle of the follicles. The effect of illness may not be noticeable until the hair developed during the period of the illness has grown above the level of the skin. Hair tends to grow slowly during illness but may grow more quickly than usual during convalescence.

Fevers, especially if body temperature rises above 39.5 °C as in pneumonia, influenza, typhoid fever and measles, may be followed by diffuse hair fall at any time up to 2 months after the illness, and abnormal hair fall may continue for about 6 weeks. This is due to the premature entry of the follicles into the resting stage (telogen) of their cycle.

Illness such as anaemia, heart disorders and some forms of cancer which affect the general blood supply can also reduce hair growth. Diffuse hair loss often follows surgical shock or the shock of a serious accident. Some drugs given to combat illness may also cause hair fall, eg. hunger-depressant drugs, anti-cancer drugs and some antibiotics.

The effect of hormones on hair growth

Hormones are chemical substances secreted directly into the blood stream from endocrine or ductless glands. The names and positions of these glands are shown in Fig. 5.2. Hormones act as chemical messengers and supplement the work of the nervous system. In general the nervous system gives a quick response to a stimulus, e.g. the movement of a muscle, whereas hormones control relatively slow processes such as growth and sexual development. Each gland secretes one or more hormones, and each hormone has a specific function. The glands and their secretions are listed in Table 5.1, which also shows the effect of the secretions on the hair and skin.

Changes in hormone level during pregnancy increase the period of anagen and bring many follicles into anagen at the same time. When oestrogen levels fall after delivery of the baby, these follicles enter

Table 5.1 Endocrine secretions and their effect on hair

Gland	Secretion	Function	Effect on hair and skin
Pituitary (in base of brain)	Growth hormone. Hormones which control other glands, e.g. adrenal, thyroid and sex glands. Melanin-stimulating hormone	Controls growth. Stimulates activity of other glands	Excess secretion causes coarsening of skin and increase in hair growth. Deficiency causes loss of hair and ageing of the skin.
Thyroid (at front of neck)	Thyroxine (an iodine compound)	Controls the general rate at which the body works	Excess secretion causes the skin to be warm and moist, with ready flushing. The hair becomes thinner in texture. Deficiency results in coarse dry skin and dry, coarse, brittle hair. There may be hair loss in the frontal region
Parathyroid (embedded in thyroid gland)	Parathyroid hormone	Controls the amount of calcium in the blood	Lack of calcium causes abnormal keratin to be produced, resulting in chronic defects of hair, skin and nails
Adrenals (lie one over each kidney)	Cortex produces corticosterone and sex hormones. Medulla secretes adrenaline	Affects the use of nutrients by the body. Prepares the body for emergency action	Excess causes growth of facial hair in women
Pancreas (lies along side the stomach)	Insulin	Controls the level of sugar in the blood. Reduced secretion causes diabetes	
Sex glands. Ovaries in female	Oestrogen	Stimulates ovaries to produce egg cells and the development of body at puberty	Ovaries and testes control growth of body hair at puberty
Testes in male	Testosterone	Stimulates sperm product- ion and the development of the body at puberty	

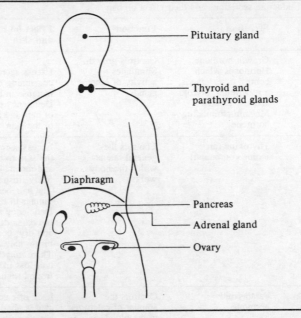

Fig 5.2 Endocrine organs (female)

catagen together, leading to an excessive loss of hair about 2 months after the birth. Similar hair fall has been reported when women stop taking oral contraceptive pills.

Hormone changes at puberty result in the growth of hair in the pubic area and the axillae, and in men on the chest and beard area. Male hormones also play a part in male pattern baldness, though age and hereditary factors are also involved.

The effect of heredity on hair growth

Certain physical characteristics such as skin and eye colour are passed on from one generation to another. The hereditary characteristics affecting hair include hair colour, the length of the periods of anagen, catagen and telogen, the amount of curl, widows peaks, white forelocks, the tendency to baldness and premature greying.

The characteristics are determined by chemical units called *genes* which are arranged in a chain along structures known as *chromosomes* contained in cell nuclei. The number of chromosomes for each species is fixed and in man each body cell contains forty-six chromosomes in its nucleus. An offspring receives twenty-three chromosomes from each of its parents.

Thus considering hair colour, a child receives a gene for colour from each of its parents. The characteristic taking precedence is known as the

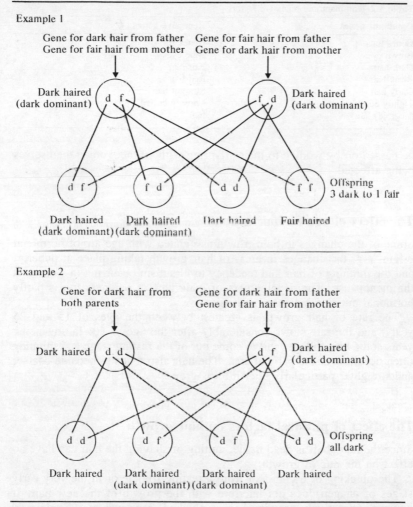

Example 1

Gene for dark hair from father   Gene for fair hair from father
Gene for fair hair from mother   Gene for dark hair from mother

Dark haired
(dark dominant)   d   f

f   d   Dark haired
(dark dominant)

d   f   f   d   d   d   f   f   Offspring
3 dark to 1 fair

Dark haired   Dark haired   Dark haired   Fair haired
(dark dominant) (dark dominant)

Example 2

Gene for dark hair from   Gene for dark hair from father
both parents   Gene for fair hair from mother

Dark haired   d   d

d   f   Dark haired
(dark dominant)

d   d   d   f   d   f   d   d   Offspring
all dark

Dark haired   Dark haired   Dark haired   Dark haired
(dark dominant) (dark dominant)

Fig 5.3 Inheritance of hair colour

dominant factor and the other as the *recessive factor*. A dark hair gene is dominant over a fair hair gene, so that if a child receives a gene for dark hair from its father and one for light hair from its mother, the gene for dark hair takes precedence and the child is dark-haired though it still carries a gene for fair hair which could be passed to the next generation. Some possible combinations showing inheritance of hair colour are shown in Fig. 5.3.

Table 5.2 shows the relative dominance of some inherited characteristics.

The tendency to baldness is hereditary and is said to be a sex-linked characteristic since it occurs only in men, though the characteristic may

Table 5.2 Dominant and recessive factors

Dominant genes	Recessive genes
Genes for:–	Genes for:–
Brown eyes	Blue eyes
Dark hair	Fair hair
Black hair	Red hair
Curly hair	Straight hair
Tightly curled	Loosely curled
(negroid) hair	hair

be passed on by women to their offspring without the women themselves being affected.

The effect of age on hair growth

Some of the changes in hair growth associated with age are of hormonal origin, e.g. the changes in areas of hair growth taking place at puberty, and the thinning of hair and tendency to hirsutism occurring in women at the menopause. The development of male pattern baldness too is partly hormonal but also increases with age.

The rate of hair growth is greatest between the ages of 15 and 25 years, and the rate slows considerably after the age of 50. In advancing years some hair follicles fail to come out of the resting stage and thinning often occurs over the parietal area. The hair also tends to become coarser and straighter particularly after it turns grey.

The effect of physical factors on hair growth

Since the hair shaft is dead tissue, cutting or shaving the hair can have no effect on the rate of growth.

The plucking of a club hair from a resting follicle or in the very early stages of anagen does not interfere with the growth of the new hair. If however an actively growing hair is plucked, regrowth may be delayed for some time to allow for repair work at the base of the follicle. The new hair usually appears within 4 to 6 weeks. Repeated pulling or traction of a hair over a period can lead to traction alopecia (see Chapter 6).

Massage of the scalp increases the blood supply to the scalp and encourages hair growth.

The effect of electro-magnetic radiations on hair growth

Ultra-violet rays stimulate cell division, so treatment by ultra-violet lamp or exposure to sunlight encourages hair growth. Hair therefore tends to grow more quickly in summer than in winter.

Infra-red rays are heat rays and exposure of the scalp to infra-red rays causes dilation of the blood vessels bringing more blood to the area, which encourages hair growth.

X-rays were at one time used for epilation (removal at the root) of scalp hairs in cases of ringworm, but this treatment has been replaced by administration of the drug griseofulvin by mouth. The dosage of radiation was carefully controlled to remove the hairs without permanent damage to the hair follicles, and hair-fall took place 14 to 21 days after treatment. The new hair sometimes underwent a change from curly to straight or vice-versa. Excessive doses of X-rays could destroy the germinal matrix, resulting in permanent baldness. The skin could also be affected, becoming wafer thin with a cracked hairless surface, and the area could become cancerous. Removal of hair by X-rays is no longer practised.

The stimulation of hair growth

If the blood supply to the scalp can be increased, more nutrients and oxygen are brought to the hair papillae and hair growth is encouraged. The circulation of blood may be increased by use of heat, massage or high frequency treatment. Since exposure to ultra-violet rays increases the rate of cell division, ultra-violet ray treatment is sometimes used to stimulate hair growth. It must be emphasised that it is impossible to prove that any treatment has been responsible for improvement in hair growth since the same growth may have taken place without treatment of any kind.

Heat treatments

Heat treatments increase blood supply to the scalp by causing dilation of the capillaries in the dermis. The treatments may be carried out by use of infra-red lamps, steamers or towels soaked in hot water.

Massage

Massage of the scalp may be carried out by hand or by the use of a vibro-massage machine. During massage the scalp is moved over the surface of the skull, the movement being possible due to the layer of very loose connective tissue attaching the scalp to the bone. Heat is produced during massage causing dilation of the blood vessels, so increasing the blood flow to the scalp. This hyperaemia increases the nutrition to the follicles and assists in the removal of waste materials from the cells. Massage is contra-indicated if septic conditions, eczema or cuts and abrasions exist on the scalp.

The movements of hand massage are as follows:

Effleurage is a stroking movement involving light pressure by the finger tips starting at the forehead and finishing at the nape. This movement is used at the beginning and end of the treatment since it has a soothing and relaxing effect.

Petrissage is the main movement of the massage and involves circular motions, with the finger tips and thumbs spread out to move the scalp over the skull in a kneading action. The fingers should be kept firmly pressed to the scalp so that there is no movement of the fingers over the scalp surface until they glide to repeat the treatment in another area. Petrissage should be carried out by use of the finger tips only because the pressure is greatest if applied to a small area.

Tapotement as used on the scalp is a vibratory movement involving a tapping action by the fingers. A small percussion appliance may be fitted on the back of the fingers and hand to make the fingers vibrate.

Vibro-massage machine

This type of machine consists of an electric motor to which a spiked rubber applicator is attached. Electric motors convert electrical energy from the mains supply into a mechanical motion which is usually a rotary action. In the case of the vibro-massage machine the motor has an eccentric cam fitted to its shaft and the applicator is mounted so that it does not rotate in a complete circle. The machine has a petrissage action on the scalp but the spiked applicator must be lifted periodically to prevent the hair from being tangled. After treatment is completed, the applicator should be sterilised in cetrimide solution and stored in a clean container.

High-frequency treatment

An electric current results from a flow of electrons. If the flow takes place in one direction only the current is a *direct current* (DC). This type of current is produced by a dry battery such as is used in a portable radio or an accumulator as in a car. If the flow of electrons changes direction periodically the current is *alternating* (AC). Mains electricity as supplied to a salon and produced by a generator at a power station is an alternating current in which the flow of electrons changes direction 100 times a second, that is it flows 50 times a second in each direction in turn and is therefore said to have a frequence (or frequency) of fifty cycles per second or 50 hertz. This is known as a *low frequency current*. In a salon high frequency apparatus, the electrons oscillate at least 1 million times a second and this is a *high frequency current*.

The high frequency apparatus has three components; the mains power supply, the oscillatory circuit producing the high frequency current, and the external circuit from which the current is applied to the client's scalp through an electrode. In older types of high frequency apparatus the oscillatory circuit involved the use of a spark gap, but later models contain valves, oscillatory tubes or transistors in electronic circuits, – possibly to be replaced in the future by a silicon chip micro-circuit.

The current of low amperage at high voltage oscillates so rapidly that when applied to the skin it does not stimulate the nerves, affect the muscles or produce electrolysis in the tissues. The energy of the oscillations is changed into heat energy in the skin causing dilation of the blood capillaries and increasing the blood flow to the area, that is it produces hyperaemia.

The current is supplied through an electrode using a round, flattened glass bulb in a rotary movement on a bald scalp, and a glass rake or comb on hairy skin. High frequency currents are sometimes applied through a bare metal electrode or 'saturator' held in the client's hand whilst the operator massages the scalp. In this case, current passes through the scalp and so to earth via the hands of the operator.

Contra-indications to the use of high frequency treatment are epilepsy, pregnancy, high blood pressure and inflammation of the skin. Metal jewellery should not be worn by the client near the area of treatment nor on the hairdresser's hands or wrists. All metal objects should be kept out of reach and alcoholic (flammable) lotions should not be applied to the scalp.

Questions

1. What is the effect of each of the following on hair growth?
   (a) shaving;   (b) plucking;   (c) age.
2. Explain what is meant by:
   (a) a holocrine gland;   (b) an endocrine gland.
   Give one example of each.
3. What is the effect of ultra-violet radiation on hair growth?
4. Name three methods by which the blood supply to the scalp could be increased.
5. How is hair growth affected by pregnancy?
6. What are the main nutrients required for hair growth?
   Describe how these nutrients reach the hair papilla from the digestive system and how they are transported to the growing cells.
7. Discuss the effect on hair, of:
   (a) a severe shortage of protein in the diet;   (b) lack of iron in the diet;   (c) an excess intake of vitamin A;   (d) lack of vitamin C.
8. Describe the structure of the scalp. Explain the movements carried out during scalp massage, and discuss the effect of each type of movement.
9. Explain why:
   (a) a tendency to baldness is called a sex-linked hereditary characteristic;
   (b) the main movement of scalp massage should be carried out using the finger tips only.
10. What precautions should be taken in the use of a high frequency apparatus?
    What conditions are contra-indicative of high-frequency treatment?

Chapter 6

Hair loss and abnormal growth

Both the loss of scalp hair and the growth of terminal hair at sites where the normal growth is of the vellus type can cause great personal distress. Recent improvements have been made in hair transplants for baldness, and the removal of abnormally growing hair is possible though the treatment is often prolonged and expensive.

A general sparseness of scalp hair (hypotrichosis) may be an inherited factor in which the total number of follicles per square centimetre is abnormally low, and the person always suffers from 'a poor head of hair'. Congenital baldness (Alopecia congenita) is rare and there is no remedy. It is due to a lack of development of the hair follicles.

Hair loss

The normal loss of about 100 scalp hairs a day is due to the growth cycle of follicles, but these hairs are usually replaced by new growth. If the rate of loss of hair exceeds new growth then either general thinning of the hair in all parts of the scalp, or baldness in patches will result. In addition to hair lost from the follicle, hair loss due to breakage of the hair by mechanical or chemical damage may take place.

General thinning of the hair (telogen effluvium)

Diffuse hair loss may be due to the disturbance of the normal hair cycle causing many follicles to enter telogen at the same time. The factors affecting the pattern of hair growth, including hair loss, were discussed in Chapter 5. The main reasons for diffuse hair loss are summarised below.
1. Changes in hormonal levels due to:
   (a) miscarriage or child birth (hair loss may take place about 2 months after delivery);
   (b) discontinuation of the use of contraceptive pills;
   (c) the menopause;
   (d) disorders of endocrine glands (especially pituitary and thyroid disorders).
2. Illnesses including:
   (a) chronic illness such as diabetes, anaemia and cancer;
   (b) illness involving high fever, e.g. typhoid, scarlet fever;

(c) the use of drugs to combat illness, e.g. anti-mitotic drugs to treat cancer.
3. Severe shock due to an accident or an operation.
4. Old age.

In the case of child birth, fevers, and shock, the hair loss is temporary and normal growth is resumed after a few months. Massage and ultra-violet treatment may encourage hair growth, though massage may appear to increase hair loss at first by removing loose telogen hairs.

Patchy hair loss

Patchy hair loss may involve:
(a) An area of skin totally devoid of hair in which case the condition is described as *alopecia*, a general term covering all types of baldness.
(b) The breaking of the hair itself, leaving an area of stubbly growth, for example in diseases such as ringworm (see Chapter 3) or in cases of mechanical or chemical damage.

Types of alopecia

Alopecia areata
Alopecia areata starts by the sudden development of small bald patches on the scalp, sometimes following the line of branches of the ophthalmic branch of the fifth cranial nerve (Trigeminal). The condition is considered to be of nervous origin and often follows shock or worry, but there is also

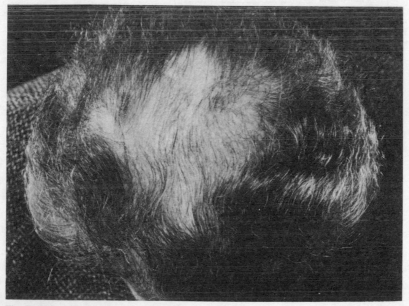

Fig 6.1 Alopecia areata

an inherited tendency towards alopecia as well. The bald patch or patches appear rapidly and are totally devoid of hair, unlike the broken-off hair of ringworm. At first the patches are usually round but if the condition spreads they may become oval, and in some cases the patches join to form larger areas of baldness (see Fig. 6.1). The skin of the patch is pale and glossy and there is no itching or inflammation. Characteristic of an increasing area of baldness are *exclamation mark hairs*. These are about half a centimetre in length and have a brush-like tip above the surface of the skin, pigment and thickness decreasing from the tip to scalp end of the hair (see Fig. 6.2).

If the hair is removed from the follicle the atrophied white bulb gives the hair the appearance of an exclamation mark. It is thought that the hair first breaks off and the stump is pushed out of the follicle when the follicle enters telogen (see Fig. 6.3).

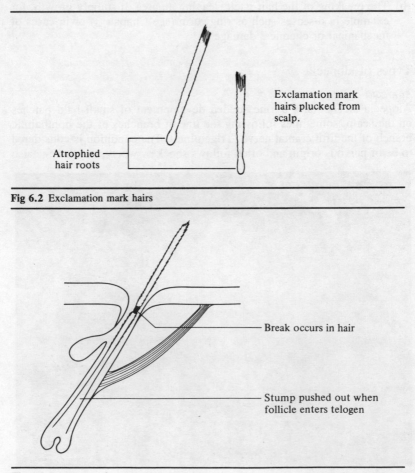

Exclamation mark hairs plucked from scalp.

Atrophied hair roots

Fig 6.2 Exclamation mark hairs

Break occurs in hair

Stump pushed out when follicle enters telogen

Fig 6.3 Formation of exclamation mark hair

The patches often clear without treatment, regrowth commencing after 2 or 3 months, but the condition may recur in times of stress. Regrowth may at first be finer than usual and the hair is sometimes white, though normal growth appears later.

If regrowth does not take place within a few months medical treatment is required and often takes the form of injecting the area with steroids. If the patches increase in size so that the whole scalp is involved and no hair remains, the condition is known as Alopecia totalis. If hair is lost from all parts of the body the condition is Alopecia universalis but this is fortunately rare.

Traction alopecia

Any treatment of the hair which involves frequent traction or pulling of the hair shafts may lead to hair breakage or the loosening of the hair in the follicle, causing traction alopecia (see Fig 6.4)

The front margin of the hair line may recede if the hair is constantly pulled back into a pony tail or bun. Tight plaiting sometimes results in traction alopecia at the base of the plait and the constant use of hairpieces may cause alopecia at the point of attachment. Traction alopecia may also be caused by over-vigorous use of nylon brushes, the use of brush rollers to obtain a tight curl, and excessive combing during the heated comb process of hair straightening. The baldness may become permanent if traction is carried out over a long period.

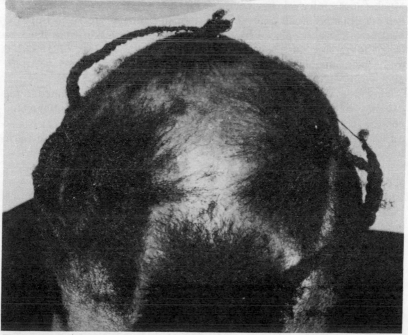

Fig 6.4 Traction alopecia

Male pattern baldness (androgenic alopecia)

In males, a tendency to baldness is a sex-linked inherited characteristic but the level of male sex hormones (androgens) and age also affect the onset of baldness. Ninety-five per cent of all male baldness is of this type. The tendency may be inherited from either or both parents for although women do not normally develop this type of baldness due to their low level of androgens, they can pass on the appropriate gene. Androgens cause the growing phase (anagen) of the hair to become progressively shorter.

The hair loss is symmetrical, starting at the front margins and receding gradually at the temples. Hair loss may also occur at the vertex and the patches may eventually join, leaving a fringe of hair over the ears and across the occipital region of the scalp where the blood supply is greatest (see Fig. 6.5 a and b).

The hair follicles in the affected area become gradually smaller and may withdraw from their blood and nerve supply. Many follicles revert to the production of a fine vellus type hair whilst in others hair growth stops completely. At the same time the sebaceous glands become much enlarged and the increased secretion of sebum leads to a shiny bald surface. Loss of hair may begin in the early twenties but starts more usually in the 30 to 40 age range and about half the men of 50 and over are bald.

Male pattern baldness cannot be prevented by any scalp treatment though it is wise to keep the scalp in as healthy a condition as possible. Much successful work has been carried out by surgeons in the field of hair transplants. Small plugs about 3 mm in diameter are taken from the bald area and are replaced by similar plugs of hairy skin from the area over the ears or the occipital region, an average number of 150–200 grafts being required. Alternatively a flap of hairy skin may be transplanted instead of the plugs.

Hair weaving is also used to overcome baldness. Hair is knotted to the existing fringe of hair, but as this grows the knotted hair needs tightening about every 6 weeks, so involving continual repeated expense. It is also difficult to clean the scalp and the tension on the existing hair can cause traction alopecia.

Senile alopecia

In old age, thinning of the hair takes place in both men and women. A diffuse hair loss known as senile alopecia occurring over the frontal area and the vertex is common.

Cicatrical alopecia

Damage to the skin with destruction of the base of the follicles always leads to permanent baldness. Burns, wounds such as severe cuts, boils which leave scar tissue, and excessive doses of X-rays, result in irregularly shaped bald patches. Cicatrical alopecia may also result from chemical burns, for example by sodium hydroxide during hair straightening if the lotion is allowed to come into contact with the skin of the scalp.

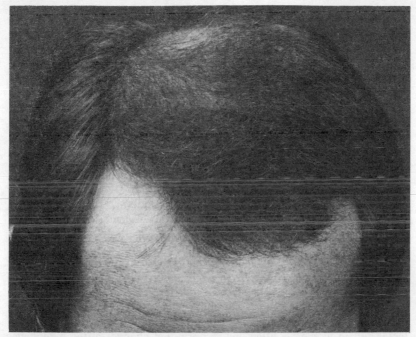

Fig 6.5(a) Male pattern of baldness (early)

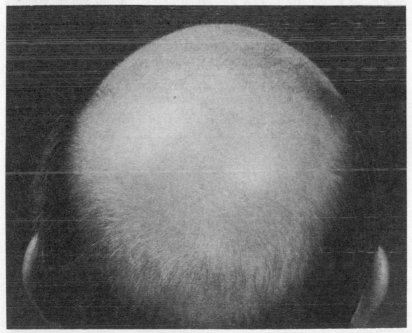

Fig 6.5(b) Male pattern of baldness (advanced)

Trichotillomania

Hair may be pulled from the follicle or broken off at skin level by nervous 'twiddling' or pulling of the hair, leaving irregular but not completely bald patches which contain some normal hairs. The condition, known as trichotillomania, is seen in some neurotic people and in some children who often find difficulty in breaking the habit.

Abnormal growth of hair

Abnormal growth of hair may take the form of the growth of terminal hair in areas where vellus hair is normally found or the hair shaft may have an unusual formation or abnormal pigmentation.

Hypertrichosis

If terminal hair grows in regions of skin normally bearing vellus type hair, the condition is known as hypertrichosis. This may be due to hormone imbalance or an inherited tendency, but often the cause is unknown. The ages at which hormonal changes are likely to affect hair growth are at puberty, the menopause and in old age. The growth of facial hair in women is often due to hormonal changes at the menopause or may be a side effect of taking certain drugs. The growth of hair in a typical masculine pattern by a female is known as *hirsutism*. Hirsutism may also be the result of a disorder such as an ovarian cyst, but in this case the hirsutism is cured when the disorder has been treated. Methods of removal of superfluous hair are considered later in this chapter.

Monilethrix

This rare hereditary condition usually occurs in infants and may disappear

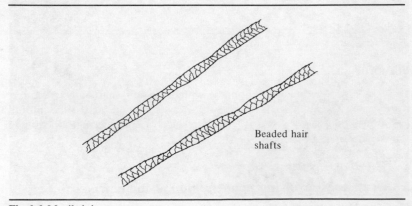

Beaded hair shafts

Fig 6.6 Monilethrix

at puberty. It may affect several members of one family but is not infectious. The hair fails to grow normally after the infant is about 6 weeks of age. Uneven rates of growth in the follicles results in the formation of beaded hair shafts, with alternate constrictions and swellings occurring periodically along the shaft (see Fig. 6.6). The hair tends to break off close to the scalp at thin parts of the shaft. Horny cones of keratin also appear at the mouths of the follicles especially in the occipital region. Treatment includes massage with vegetable oils and the removal of the keratin plugs with salicylic acid, accompanied by frequent washing. Avoidance of exposure of the hair to the sun, and gentleness in combing and brushing may enable the hair to be grown longer.

Trichonodosis

Damage to the germinal matrix of the follicle due to repeated plucking of hair or to incomplete removal of hair by electrolysis, may lead to abnormal growth in which the hair becomes knotted. One or more knots may appear in the hair shaft just above the level of the skin. The hair is usually dry with a tendency to split. Whilst appearing to be very short, the hair may actually be quite long but is looped into knots. (see Fig. 6.7).

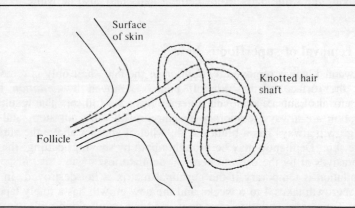

Fig 6.7 Trichonodosis

Pili torti

This is a rare hereditary condition in which the hair shafts are twisted at regular intervals along their full length. The scalp is dry and scaly and the hair brittle and easily broken. The hairs have a shimmering appearance due to the twists.

Abnormalities involving pigmentation of the hair

Ringed hair (Pili annulata). Intermittent production of melanin results in alternate bands of coloured and uncoloured areas along the hair shafts, producing ringed hair.

Leucotrichia (Poliosis). This hereditary condition involves a lack of pigment in a very localised area of the scalp, usually as a white forelock. It is a dominant characteristic so tends to appear in many generations of the same family. There is no treatment available apart from dyeing the forelock to match the remainder of the hair.

Canities (pronounced 'kanishiez'). The lack of pigment formation by the melanocytes in some follicles leads to a mixture of coloured and uncoloured hair causing greyness or canities. This is usually due to a combination of age and hereditary factors, but may also be caused by illhealth or nervous conditions. Greying before the age of 30 years is regarded as premature greying. Lack of some of the B group vitamins has been shown to be responsible for greying in rats but has not been proved to affect man. Hair often becomes coarser when greying takes place. If greying is associated with illness, colour may eventually return but this is rare. Senile greying is irreversible. Going white overnight has no scientific basis as the hair shaft is dead tissue, though it is often said to take place. If the hair is a mixture of coloured and white hairs (grey) it is possible for the coloured hairs to go into telogen through shock and fall, so leaving the white hairs. Replacement hairs may also be white.

The removal of superfluous hair

If unwanted hair is removed by *depilation* the hair shaft only is removed from the surface of the skin. If hair is removed by *epilation* both the shaft and root are removed together from the follicle. The results of depilation are always temporary as hair growth does not stop, and the new growth always has a blunt cut tip when it appears above the surface of the skin. Depilation may be brought about by shaving, cutting, the use of abrasives or by the use of chemical depilatories.

Epilation is temporary if the germinal matrix is not destroyed. In this case regrowth takes 4 to 6 weeks and the new growth has a finely tapered point. Temporary epilation may be carried out by plucking with tweezers or by waxing. Effective permanent epilation involving the destruction of the germinal matrix can be carried out by galvanic electrolysis or by diathermy. Older methods of epilation included the use of X-rays or the oral administration of thallium salts. These methods were used to remove hair in cases of ringworm before the introduction of the drug griseofulvin.

Bleaching is sometimes a suitable alternative to hair removal for soft dark hairs on the face since blonde hair is less noticeable than dark hair. One part of oil bleach to 2 parts of 6 per cent hydrogen peroxide is suitable for this purpose, though in some cases there may be irritation of the skin. Repeated bleaching weakens the hair and gives it a tendency to break.

Methods of depilation

Abrasion may be carried out by the use of pumice stone or by abrasive emery gloves. The method is most suitable for the arms and legs which should be well lathered with soap before treatment. The hair is worn away from the skin mechanically by friction. Too vigorous rubbing may cause skin irritation and an emollient cream should be used afterwards.

Shaving is satisfactory for underarm hair but not for female facial hair, for although the texture and colour is not affected by shaving, the new growth may feel more bristly as it is less flexible than longer hair and will be blunt cut, not tapered as in the case of an uncut hair.

Cutting has a similar effect to shaving and is suitable for hair growing from a mole, since the plucking of such hairs should be avoided (see Chapter 3).

Chemical depilatories are substances which break down the chemical structure of keratin. They consist of alkaline reducing agents which cause the hair fibres to swell, break the cystine linkages and finally destroy the polypeptide chains themselves. Modern depilatories are mostly creams containing 3–4 per cent of calcium thioglycollate and sufficient calcium hydroxide to give a pH of about 12. The high pH lessens the time required for hair removal. Since the cream could also break down skin keratin, a test on a small area of skin should be made before full application to avoid the possibility of skin irritation.

These depilatories are suitable for removal of underarm hair and for the arms and legs. They should be used with great care on the more sensitive skin of the face. The creams should not be left on any skin longer than the manufacturers' recommended time or the surface layer of skin may be damaged. The recommended time is calculated so that hair removal takes place with the minimum of skin damage.

Older types of chemical depilatories contained sodium or barium sulphide solutions. These had a most unpleasant smell of bad eggs due to the formation of hydrogen sulphide gas and were too drastic on the skin.

After application of chemical depilatories for underarm hair removal, the use of deodorants or antiperspirants should be avoided for at least 24 hours. Contra-indications to the use of chemical depilatories are sensitive areas of skin, skin blemishes and skin infections.

Methods of epilation

Plucking
Plucking with tweezers is suitable for isolated hairs such as eyebrows.

Waxing
This is a form of mass plucking of hairs. A blend of beeswax and paraffin wax, or beeswax and resin, having a melting point just above normal skin temperature is suitable. The waxes are melted by warming and are then applied to the skin and allowed to solidify. When the wax is stripped off

quickly in the opposite direction to the growth of hairs epilation takes place, the hairs becoming embedded in the wax.

A thermostatically controlled pan is often used for warming the wax to avoid overheating and the possibility of fire, and also to prevent skin burns. After treatment the wax is melted and filtered to remove loose hairs before re-use.

Contra-indications to waxing are skin infections, cuts, abrasions, moles and sensitive or sunburnt skin. Waxing is usually carried out on the arms and legs but can be used for facial hair.

Electrolysis

Tissue fluid in the skin is a salty solution, the salts, chiefly sodium chloride, being split into electrically charged particles or *ions*. These ions enable the solution to conduct an electric current, and such a solution is known as an *electrolyte*. In solution, sodium chloride forms two separate ions. One (*the cation*) is a positively charged sodium ion and the other (*the anion*) is a negatively charged chloride ion.

If two platinum plates or *electrodes* are immersed in a sodium chloride solution and are connected to a battery providing a direct electric current, the movement of the ions in the electrolyte completes the circuit (see

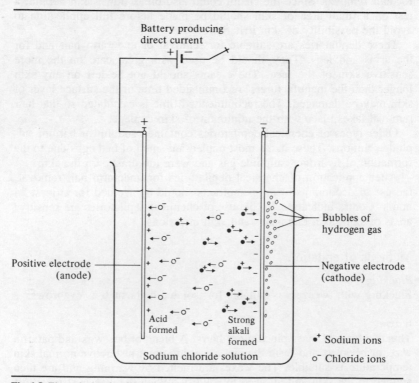

Fig 6.8 Electrolysis of sodium chloride solution

Fig. 6.8). The electrodes become charged according to their battery connection. One, *the anode*, becomes positively charged and attracts the negatively charged chloride ions. The other, *the cathode*, becomes negatively charged and attracts the positively charged sodium ions.

Chemical changes take place at the electrodes as follows:

At the anode the chloride ions lose their charges, chlorine is formed and reacts with the water to produce hydrochloric and hypochlorous acids.

At the cathode the sodium ions receive a negative charge from the electrode and form sodium atoms which react with water to produce sodium hydroxide, and hydrogen gas.

The chemical changes which occur when a current passes through an electrolyte are called *electrolysis*.

In hair removal by electrolysis the cathode is a fine platinum needle, insulated except for the very tip. The needle is carefully inserted between the inner and outer root sheaths to reach the base of the follicle (see Fig. 6.9).

The anode is a sponge soaked in sodium chloride solution and is applied to the surface of the skin. A very small current of not more than 3 milliamps is required. The same chemical reactions as described for the electrolysis of sodium chloride take place. At the cathode, sodium hydroxide (a caustic alkali) is produced and this destroys the germinal matrix

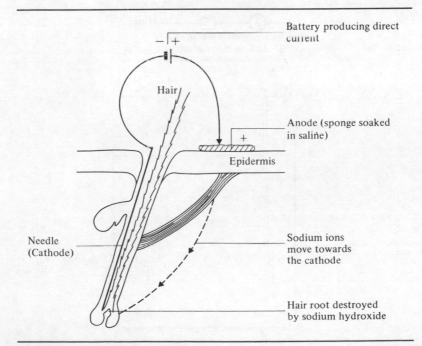

Battery producing direct current

Hair

Anode (sponge soaked in saline)

Epidermis

Needle
(Cathode)

Sodium ions move towards the cathode

Hair root destroyed by sodium hydroxide

Fig 6.9 Removal of hair by electrolysis

of the follicle, so that regrowth of hair is prevented. The reaction takes about 40 seconds and is known to be completed when bubbles of hydrogen gas rise up the follicle. The current should then be switched off and the hair gently removed with tweezers. The method has been satisfactorily used for many years but is now mostly superseded by diathermy since more hairs can be removed per session and the process is less painful than electrolysis. Because of the difficulty of placing the needle in the exact position in the hair follicle, regrowth in a proportion of follicles is always to be expected.

Experiment 6.1 Electrolysis

Using the apparatus and circuit shown in Fig. 6.10, observe and note any changes that occur at the electrodes whilst an electric current is passing through each of the following liquids:

(a) liquid paraffin;
(b) de-ionised water;
(c) tap water;
(d) acidified tap water;
(e) sodium chloride solution.

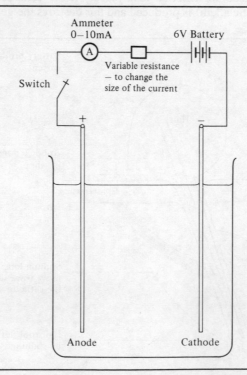

Fig 6.10 Apparatus for experiment on electrolysis

Diathermy

Diathermy, or electro-coagulation, is sometimes incorrectly referred to as electrolysis, but in diathermy the destruction of the germinal matrix is by heat, and not by the chemical changes due to the passage of electricity through the skin. A platinum diathermy needle, insulated except at its tip, carries the current both to and from the base of the follicle. The needle is inserted into the follicle before the current is switched on. The current used in diathermy is a high frequency alternating current (see Chapter 5) which produces heat in the tissues at the point of the needle. The heat coagulates the protein in the cells of the hair matrix, so destroying them. A hair can be epilated in 1–2 seconds by this method and up to 100 hairs can be removed in an hour.

Surgical methods of hair removal

Groups of hairs may be removed by surgical operation. A flap of skin is cut back and the bases of the hair follicles removed before the skin is restored to its original position. This is a very satisfactory method and can be performed without permanent scarring.

Photo-epilation

The most modern method of epilation is by use of a *laser beam*. The germinal matrix of the follicle is destroyed by a very fine but intense beam of single frequency light consisting of uniform pulses, which is accurately concentrated on to the required area.

Questions

1. What is the cause of:
   (a) canities;   (b) ringed hair;   (c) trichonodosis?
2. Which hair conditions are associated with the following?
   (a) exclamation mark hairs;   (b) beaded hair shafts;
   (c) a white forelock.
3. Explain the difference between epilation and depilation. Name a chemical often used in modern depilatories.
4. Briefly describe the following terms:
   (a) alopecia areata;   (b) alopecia totalis;   (c) traction alopecia.
5. Explain how the hair becomes weakened and subject to fracture in each of the following cases:
   (a) tinea capitis;   (b) trichotillomania;   (c) monilethrix.
6. What advice would you give to a young female client
   (a) complaining of severe hair loss a few months after child birth;   (b) with a patch of dark hairs growing under her chin;   (c) who is worried about premature greying;   (d) who complains of the development of small areas of baldness on the scalp?

7. Discuss the causes and progress of male pattern baldness. What methods are available for overcoming the problem of hair loss?
8. Discuss the possible causes of a diffuse loss of scalp hair.
9. What is meant by hypertrichosis? What is the usual cause and what methods of treatment are available for this condition?
10. What may be the effect of
    (a) sodium hydroxide applied to the hair;   (b) frequent tight plaiting of hair;   (c) the use of X-rays on the scalp;   (d) chemical depilatories left on the skin beyond the recommended time.

Chapter 7

The formulation of hairdressing products

Products for use on the hair seldom consist of single chemical elements or even single chemical compounds, but are usually complex mixtures of compounds in the form of *solutions* or *emulsions*. The product must have a suitable viscosity (thickness) and be of a suitable strength for its purpose.

Careful testing of products is carried out by manufacturers to avoid damage to the hair, skin, eyes or to the general health of the user. When stored under normal conditions, the product must not deteriorate during its expected shelf-life and, in order to be acceptable in use, must have both a pleasant appearance and a pleasant odour.

Most containers of hairdressing products are now labelled in litres or millilitres according to the volume of their contents, though cubic centimetres may be used. Shampoo, for example, may be purchased in bulk by the litre, whilst small bottles of setting lotion or tubes of dye designed for individual use, are usually marked in millilitres.

A millilitre (ml) is a thousandth part of a litre (l)

or   1 litre = 1000 ml

A litre is also equal to a thousand cubic centimetres (cm³)

or   1 litre = 1000 cm³

A cubic centimetre has the same volume as a small cube with sides one centimetre in length. For practical purposes a cubic centimetre and a millilitre can be regarded as equivalent.

Solutions

The solutions used in many hairdressing products consist of one or more *solutes* dissolved in either a single *solvent* or a mixture of solvents. Many additives to the basic solution may be included to improve the performance and appearance of the product. All the additives must, of course, be soluble in the solvent used. The commonest and cheapest solvent is water, but where the required solute is insoluble in water or where water must be avoided, for example in lacquers and other products designed for use on dry hair after setting, other solvents such as various forms of alcohol (ethanol, isopropanol or industrial methylated spirit) must be used. Examples of solutions used in hairdressing products are listed in Table 7.1.

Table 7.1 Solutions

Product (solution)	Active ingredient (Solute)	Solvents	Additives
Shampoo (liquid)	15% triethanolamine lauryl sulphate (TLS)	Water	Foam booster conditioner colour, perfume
Acid rinse lemon vinegar	10% citric acid 5% acetic acid	Water Water	
Conditioning rinse	1–1.5% cetrimide	Water	Cetyl alcohol (thickener)
After-shave lotion	menthol	Industrial methylated spirit (IMS)	Perfume cetrimide (antiseptic)
Setting lotion	1% gum tragacanth or 2% plastic resin	Water and isopropanol IMS and water	Plasticisers, borax, preservative Plasticiser
Hair lacquer	8% shellac or 4% plastic resin	IMS and water IMS	Plasticiser Plasticiser
Liquid - brilliantine	15% castor oil	IMS	Perfume
Heat perm lotion	2% sodium sulphite 20% ammonium hydroxide	Water	Borax
Cold wave lotion	6–10% ammonium thioglycollate	Water	Ammonium hydroxide
Neutraliser	6% hydrogen peroxide or 5% sodium bromate	Water Water	Shampoo (thickener) Shampoo (thickener)
Bleach (liquid)	6% hydrogen peroxide	Water	Ammonium hydroxide and shampoo
Temporary dye	azo dye	Water	Citric or tartaric acid
Semi-permanent dyes	nitro dyes	Benzyl alcohol and water	Methyl cellulose (thickener)

Product (solution)	Active ingredient (Solute)	Solvents	Additives
Oxidation dyes (liquid type)	para dyes	Isopropanol and water	Ammonium hydroxide sodium sulphite
Nail enamel	12% nitrocellulose 6% formaldehyde resin	Ethyl acetate	Plasticiser silicone fluid

Solutions are usually thin clear liquids which would not easily stay in position on the hair. It is therefore often convenient to increase the viscosity of a solution by addition of a thickener. Various substances such as methyl cellulose, gums and alkanolamides (non-ionic detergents) may be used for this purpose. Clear liquid shampoos of the triethanolamine lauryl sulphate type may be thickened by the addition of either soaps or common salt (sodium chloride). Neutralisers for use in cold waving are sometimes whipped up into a foam with sodium lauryl sulphate shampoo to keep them in place in the hair, and semi-permanent dyes are often thickened by methyl cellulose.

Experiment 7.1   The thickening of soapless shampoo
Using a 10 per cent solution of TLS, prepare four test-tubes each containing 50 ml of solution. Keep one tube as a control. To each of the others add increasing quantities of sodium chloride, e.g. 0.5 g to the first tube; 1 g to the second; and 2 g to the third. Note the effect on the viscosity of the shampoo. The viscosity increases to a maximum and then decreases and the shampoo then becomes thinner as more salt is added. A thick shampoo does not, therefore, necessarily indicate that it is concentrated.

The strength of solutions

The strength or concentration of a solution often determines its use and this is usually expressed as a percentage of solute in the solution. The percentage may be expressed by weight as the number of grammes of solute in 100 g of solution, or by volume as the number of millilitres of solute in 100 ml of solution. Thus a 30 per cent solution contains 30 parts by weight or volume of solute in 100 parts by weight or volume of solution. The parts must always be measured in the same units. A 30 per cent solution containing 30 g of solute in 100 g of solution would be prepared by dissolving 30 g of solute in 70 g of solvent to make 100 g of solution.

Hairdressers may purchase shampoo in concentrated liquid form which requires dilution with water before use. Instructions for dilution vary, and may be in the form for example that '1 litre makes 5 litres', in which case 1 litre of concentrate must be added to 4 litres of water. Alternatively the instruction may be 'use a 1 in 8 solution' which requires 1 part of concentrate to 7 parts of water, both measured by volume.

Different strengths of shampoo may be used for different types of hair. For example,

Hair type	Triethanolamine lauryl sulphate (%)	Water (%)
dry	10	90
normal	20	80
greasy	50	50

Similarly, when perming, the strength of lotion must be related to the type of hair on which it is to be used.

For example,

Percentage of ammonium thioglycollate in perm lotion:

10   per cent for virgin hair which would be resistant to perming;

 8   per cent for normal hair;

 5   per cent for tinted or very porous hair.

Some substances are used for quite different purposes at different concentrations.

For example,

1. Salicylic acid (hydroxybenzoic acid):
   (a) Traces may be added to hairdressing products as a preservative;
   (b) 0.1 per cent solution is used as a stabiliser for hydrogen peroxide;
   (c) 3 per cent solution is used in keratolytic preparations for removal of dandruff scale;
   (d) 12 per cent solutions are used as corn removers.
2. Sodium hydroxide (caustic soda):
   (a) 2 per cent solutions are used as nail cuticle removers;
   (b) 5 per cent solutions are used in chemical hair straighteners;
   (c) 10–15 per cent solutions are used to free drains from blockage by hair.

The strength of solution is important since, above certain concentrations, some solutions may be damaging to the skin or hair, e.g. cetrimide is used in conditioning rinses but in concentrations above 2 per cent it is damaging to the eyes, causing permanent opacity of the cornea (the clear outer covering at the front of the eyeball). Even at low concentrations sodium hydroxide is caustic and will burn the skin. Hydrogen peroxide at concentrations above 9 per cent (30 vol) will also burn the skin and damage the hair.

Experiment 7.2   Effect of sodium hydroxide on hair

Place a weft of hair in each of the following solutions of sodium hydroxide 2 per cent solution, 5 per cent solution and 15 per cent solution. Compare speed and extent of hair damage.

(WARNING: sodium hydroxide burns the skin.)

The strength of hydrogen peroxide solution may be expressed as a *percentage strength* or as a *volume strength*. Percentage strength is the number of grammes of hydrogen peroxide in 100 g of solution, so that a 3 per cent solution contains 3 g of hydrogen peroxide and therefore 97 g of water in 100 g of solution. When heated or in the presence of catalysts, hydrogen peroxide readily gives off oxygen gas. Volume strength is the number of parts of oxygen gas measured by volume, which can be obtained from one part of hydrogen peroxide. Thus a 10 volume solution of hydrogen peroxide will give off 10 parts of oxygen from 1 part of the hydrogen peroxide; or 1 ml of 10 volume hydrogen peroxide gives 10 ml of free oxygen.

As 1 ml of 3 per cent solution of hydrogen peroxide also gives off 10 ml of free oxygen, a 3 per cent solution has the same strength as a 10 volume solution. The percentage strengths corresponding to other volume strengths may be calculated by proportion. Hydrogen peroxide is normally available in the following strengths which are used as indicated below.

3 per cent (10 vol) used in brightening rinses
6 per cent (20 vol) for bleaching, 'neutralising' cold perms, oxidation
                     of permanent dyes
9 per cent (30 vol) for tinting lighter
12 per cent (40 vol) for bleached tips and streaking
18 per cent (60 vol) ⎫ used only as stock solutions for dilution, and
30 per cent (100 vol) ⎭ must never be used on the hair or skin undiluted

Different strengths of hydrogen peroxide have different relative densities (specific gravities). For example,

the relative density of 30 per cent (100 vol) hydrogen peroxide is 1.110
            and that of 6 per cent (20 vol) hydrogen peroxide is 1.020

As hydrogen peroxide is increasingly diluted its relative density approaches that of pure water which is 1.

The relative density of a liquid may be measured by the use of a hydrometer which is floated in the liquid, when the relative density may be read directly at surface level on the scale in the stem of the instrument. Special hydrometers known as peroxometers are available to measure the strength of hydrogen peroxide solution, the value of the relative density being replaced on the scale by the corresponding percentage strength or the volume strength of the hydrogen peroxide.

Alcohols used as solvents

Alcohols form a series of organic compounds, the names of which all end in '-ol'. They contain a hydroxyl group, but are not alkalis since they do not ionise, and no hydroxyl ions are formed.

Ethanol is often referred to simply as 'alcohol' and is the type of alcohol contained in alcoholic drinks. In its pure state its production and sale are strictly controlled by law, and in hairdressing products it is more often used in its denatured form of **industrial methylated spirit**. This contains 95 per cent of ethanol together with 5 per cent of a more poisonous type of alcohol called **methanol**, which renders industrial methylated spirit unfit to drink. For household purposes methylated spirit is coloured purple by the addition of a dye.

Isopropanol has a less pleasant smell than ethanol or methylated spirit but is cheaper and is sometimes used for cleaning windows and mirrors. Isopropanol, ethanol and industrial methylated spirit are all colourless, highly flammable liquids which will mix with water. They are all used as solvents for hair lacquers and setting lotions.

Benzyl alcohol is used in semi-permanent dyes as a dispersing agent. The solvent separates or disperses clusters of dye molecules, easing their entry into the hair shaft.

Colloidal solutions

The solutions of certain substances such as starches and soaps are cloudy, and contain particles which are larger than those of the solute in a true solution, yet are small enough to pass through a filter paper. This type of solution, which remains cloudy even after filtering, is known as a colloidal solution or a colloid. If the colloid is very concentrated, a gel (a semi-solid jelly) is produced. A soap gel is formed if a hot concentrated solution of soap is cooled, and soft soap shampoos often take this form.

Emulsions

Emulsions are milky liquids or creams consisting of droplets of one liquid suspended in another liquid. The two liquids must be insoluble in each other and are therefore *immiscible* (i.e. they cannot be mixed). Emulsions thus consist of two phases, the droplets forming the *disperse phase* and the liquid in which they are suspended forming the *continuous phase* (see Fig. 7.1).

An emulsion may be formed by shaking the two liquids together, but unless a third substance known as the *emulsifying agent* is present the liquids tend to separate quickly into two layers. Emulsifying agents are substances which are partially soluble in both the liquids of the emulsion, and so form a bridge between the two by surrounding the suspended droplets, preventing them from coalescing, and thus make the emulsion permanent.

Most common emulsions are mixtures of oil and water. Droplets of oil suspended in water form an *oil-in-water* (O/W) emulsion, whilst droplets of water suspended in oil form a *water-in-oil* (W/O) emulsion. The type of emulsion formed depends on the emulsifying agent and not on the proportions of oil and water present. Examples of substances used as emulsifying agents are detergents (soaps, soapless and cationic), synthetic emulsifying waxes such as Lanette wax, and beeswax with borax. The substance in which the emulsifying agent is most soluble normally forms the continuous phase.

If the two phases have very different densities *'creaming'* may take

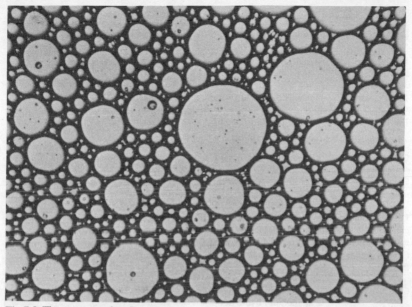

Fig 7.1 The structure of an Emulsion

place as the disperse phase rises or falls in the continuous phase (like the cream in milk). Such an emulsion is easily restored by shaking.

Cracking of an emulsion occurs if the droplets of the disperse phase coalesce, in which case the emulsion cannot be restored by shaking. In emulsion type perm lotions it is important that the emulsion is very stable, since if cracking occurred oil would be deposited on the hair, which would then prevent the penetration of the active ingredients. On the other hand hair control creams should crack immediately on contact with the hair or the white cream would remain visible on the hair.

In general, oil-in-water emulsions are preferred in hairdressing preparations as they are less greasy than water-in-oil types, since the oil is always surrounded by the water of the continuous phase. Oil-in-water emulsions are easily diluted with water and may be washed off the skin and hair by water alone. Water-in-oil emulsions do not rinse off easily and must be washed away by use of a detergent. Examples of emulsions used in hairdressing and manicure products are listed in Table 7.2.

In making emulsions the ingredients of the two phases must be heated separately to 70 °C, the emulsifying agent being added to either phase. Substances soluble in oil such as waxes and lanolin may be added to the oil phase before heating, and substances soluble in water such as glycerol, cetrimide (antiseptic), ammonium thioglycollate (in perm lotion) and gums (used for thickening the water phase to prevent creaming) may be added to the water phase before heating. The two phases are then mixed at 70 °C and stirred until cool. Perfume and any other volatile substances must be added when the emulsion has cooled to 40 °C.

Table 7.2 Emulsions

Product	Main ingredients	Emulsifying agent	Type of emulsion
Brushless shaving cream	mineral oil, lanolin and water	Triethanolamine soap	O/W
Hand cream	lanolin, glycerol, water	Lanette wax	O/W
Barrier cream	liquid paraffin, lanolin, silicone oils, water	Lanette wax	O/W
Cuticle cream	mineral oil and water	Beeswax/borax	W/O
Conditioning rinse	cetrimide, mineral oil, lanolin and water	Cetrimide cetyl alcohol	O/W
Dressing-out cream	mineral oil and water	Triethanolamine soap	O/W
Control cream (men's)	mineral oil and water	Beeswax/borax	W/O
Cold wave lotion	ammonium thioglycollate, ammonium hydroxide, mineral oil and water	Cetyl alcohol	O/W
Hair straightener	ammonium thioglycollate, ammonium hydroxide, mineral oil and water	Glyceryl monostearate	O/W

Experiment 7.3   Preparation of a cationic conditioner

Ingredients: Oil phase	– lanolin	2 g
	mineral oil	2 g
	cetyl alcohol (hexadecanol)	10 g
Water phase	– cetrimide	1 g
	deionised water	85 ml

Heat the lanolin, mineral oil and cetyl alcohol to 70 °C on a water bath. Dissolve the cetrimide in the water and heat the solution to 70 °C. Pour the water mixture gradually into the oil mixture, stirring all the time until the emulsion cools. Perfume may then be added if desired. Do not exceed the amount of cetrimide in the cream as higher concentrations are dangerous to the eyes.

Oils, fats and waxes used in hairdressing products

1. Animal and vegetable oils, fats and waxes
(a) Animal fats, e.g. beef and mutton fat, are used in soap manufacture;
(b) Vegetable oils, e.g. palm oil, castor oil and coconut oil, are used in the manufacture of soap, soapless detergents, control creams and brilliantines;

(c) Waxes such as beeswax, spermaceti wax (from whales) and carnauba wax (from the surface of palm leaves), are used in control creams. Lanolin, which is obtained by washing sheep wool, is similar to sebum and contains a mixture of waxes and fatty acids. It is used as a hair and skin conditioner and may be added to shampoos, lacquer, conditioning creams and hand creams.

All the above oils, fats and waxes are members of a class of organic compounds known as *esters*. Simple esters are sweet-smelling liquids, e.g. amyl acetate (smells of pear drops) and ethyl acetate, both of which are used as solvents for nail enamel. They are formed by the reaction between an organic acid and an alcohol.

organic acid + alcohol = an ester + water

e.g. acetic acid + ethanol = ethyl acetate + water

Animal and vegetable oils, fats and waxes are more complex types of ester. The oils and fats are esters of complex acids such as stearic acid, oleic acid and lauric acid, and an alcohol called glycerol. One molecule of glycerol reacts with three molecules of acid to make a molecule of fat or oil, so these esters are known also as *triglycerides*. Oils are normally liquid at room temperature whilst at that temperature fats are solid.

fatty acid + glycerol = an oil (triglyceride) + water

e.g. lauric acid + glycerol = glyceryl laurate (ester) + water
(coconut oil)

Waxes are esters of similar acids with complex alcohols other than glycerol.

fatty acid + complex alcohol = a wax + water

e.g. lauric acid + cetyl alcohol = cetyl laurate + water
(spermaceti wax)

Mineral oils and waxes
Petroleum, which is found in the ground, is the source of mineral oils and waxes. These substances are not esters but are hydrocarbons consisting only of the elements carbon and hydrogen. Petroleum products may be separated by means of distillation. In addition to petrol and gases which are used for heating purposes, petroleum products include liquid paraffin, soft paraffin or petroleum jelly (Vaseline) and paraffin wax. These products may all be used in control creams and brilliantines.

Synthetic oils and waxes
(a) *Silicone oils* (silicone fluids) contain dimethyl silicone, a polymer which consists of long chains of silicon and oxygen atoms with methyl groups attached at regular intervals. This structure enables

silicones to form a thin layer over a surface, the film being strongly *water-repellent*. Silicones are thus incorporated into barrier creams to leave a water-repellent film on the skin. In hairdressing products a similar water-resistant barrier on the hair makes them useful in lacquers and setting lotions. They are particularly useful in setting lotions for blow drying as the film is *heat resistant*. Silicone emulsions are used as hair-straightening agents for heated comb methods, the smooth surface given to the hair lessening the possibility of mechanical damage. They may also be used as conditioners in shampoos and have an antistatic and softening effect.

(b) *Synthetic emulsifying waxes*, e.g. Lanette wax, are mixtures of cetyl alcohol (hexadecanol) and stearyl alcohol (octadecanol). They are used in the preparation of emulsion creams.

The pH of the product

The pH scale

The acidity or alkalinity of a substance may be measured on the pH scale of 0–14 (see Table 7.3). At a pH of 7, the *neutral point* of the scale, substances are neither alkaline nor acid. Values below 7 indicate acidity (the lower the number, the stronger the acid) whilst values 7–14 indicate increasing alkalinity. The pH value of a substance may be determined electrically using a pH meter, or more simply but less accurately by the colour change of a pH paper (universal indicator paper) dipped into a solution of the substance. The colour of the paper has then to be compared with the manufacturer's chart relating colour to the numerical pH value.

All acids contain the element hydrogen and in solution give rise to hydrogen ions (H^+) which carry a positive electrical charge. The quantity of hydrogen ions produced by an acid or the hydrogen ion concentration determines its pH value. Alkalis always give rise to negatively charged hydroxyl ions (OH^-). Pure water is neutral because it contains equal quantities of hydrogen ions and hydroxyl ions. The actual quantity of hydrogen ions in pure water is very small, only one ten-millionth of a gramme in 1 litre, i.e. $\dfrac{1}{10\,000\,000}$ or $\dfrac{1}{10^7}$ grammes per litre. On the pH scale a hydrogen ion concentration of $\dfrac{1}{10^7}$ is represented by 7, which is the logarithm of 10^7. A solution of pH 6 contains $\dfrac{1}{10^6}$ grammes or one-millionth of a gramme per litre which is ten times more than in a solution of pH 7. Thus because the pH scale is logarithmic each number on the scale is 10 times greater or smaller than the adjacent numbers. A solution of pH 3 is ten times more strongly acid than one of pH 4 and ten times less acid than one of pH 2. Similarly a solution of pH 9 is ten times more alkaline than one of pH 8 and ten times less alkaline than one of pH 10.

Table 7.3 The pH scale

Hairdressing products	Strength of acid or alkali	pH value	Typical colour change (pH paper)	Effect on hair, skin and eyes
	Very strong acid			
			Red	
		1		Hair hardened and becomes stringy
		2		Hydrogen bonds and salt linkages broken in hair
	Strong acid			
		3	Orange	
				Burns skin
		4		
Acetic acid rinse Citric acid rinse Acid dyes		5	Yellow	Conditioning effect on cuticle scales
Skin secretions	Weak acid			
Ammonium sulphite (perm lotions)		6		Stings eyes
Pure water Soapless shampoos	Neutral	7	Green	
Triethanolamine soaps				
		8		Stings eyes
Other soaps	Weakly alkaline			Roughens cuticle
Nitro dyes Oil bleach Cold wave lotion Permanent dyes		9	Light blue	Hair begins to swell and becomes more porous Hair damage
		10		Hydrogen bonds and salt linkages broken Burns skin
	Strongly alkaline	11		Disulphide linkages broken
Hair straighteners			Dark blue	Hair destroyed polypeptide chains broken
Depilatories		12		
		13		
	Very strongly alkaline		Violet	
		14		

In the same way a pH of 11 indicates a liquid which is 100 times more alkaline than one of pH 9.

The importance of pH

The pH of hairdressing products is important because of the effect of acids and alkalis on hair, skin and the eyes. In general alkalis are more damaging to keratin than are acids. Strong alkalis will completely destroy hair whilst strong acids make hair harsh and stringy without destroying the fibre. Hair may be permanently damaged if the pH of a product exceeds 9.5. Weak alkalis soften hair, make it swell and cause roughening of the cuticle scales. They are often added to hairdressing products for this purpose to make the hair more porous and thus enable other chemicals to enter the hair shaft. Therefore perm lotions, bleaches and permanent dyes are usually made alkaline by the addition of ammonium hydroxide, to assist the penetration of the main ingredients into the hair. Setting lotions may also be made alkaline, usually by the addition of borax, to soften the hair as an aid in setting. The use of alkalis thus tends to leave hair in poor condition.

Weak acids, such as acetic or citric acid, make hair smoother by decreasing swelling and causing the cuticle scales to become more compact. Thus treatment by weak acids has a conditioning effect on hair. Sebum, which is spread along the hair shaft by brushing, is slightly acid so the surface of the hair is normally in a slightly acid state.

Both strong acids and strong alkalis will burn the skin, and strong mineral acids have no place in hairdressing products. The most alkaline product is hair-straightening cream which contains sodium hydroxide and has a pH of about 12. This must be kept off the skin so the scalp is normally protected by petroleum jelly before straightening takes place, and a backwash basin must be used when washing the straightener from the hair. Depilatories containing calcium thioglycollate also have a pH of 12, and contact time on the skin should be kept to a minimum or the upper layers of the epidermis may be removed. Cold wave lotions of pH 9.5 can burn the skin usually causing mild erythema. The use of alkaline soaps of pH 8–9 has little effect on the skin since they are usually quickly rinsed away, and the normal skin secretions soon restore the slight acidity of the skin surface.

Weak acids and weak alkalis both cause stinging of the eyes. Neutral shampoos are the most satisfactory, but many detergents used in shampoos cause eye irritation and care should always be taken to avoid the entry of any hairdressing products into the client's eyes.

Acid-balanced products

Many modern products are 'acid balanced' or 'pH balanced', that is they have a pH of about 5, approximating to that of the skin secretions in the acid mantle. Acid-balanced products are designed to maintain this pH and to avoid damage to the hair by products which are too alkaline. Acid-balanced products include shampoos, conditioners, setting lotions and lacquers. Similarly acid or neutral cold wave lotions have been developed which rely on heat instead of alkalis to aid penetration of the lotions. The heat also increases the speed of the chemical reactions taking place in the hair. Acid products are also used in treatments following alkaline cold waves, bleaches and permanent colours to neutralise any remaining alkalinity.

Buffering

In order that a product may maintain the same pH during its shelf-life, the product may be buffered. Substances called *buffers* are added during manufacture and will prevent slight changes in acidity or alkalinity, so maintaining the product at the desired pH. For example cream bleaches are buffered by the addition of urea peroxide or butyl peroxide. The presence of ammonium thioglycollate and ammonium hydroxide in perm lotion forms a buffered solution but ammonium chloride is often added as an additional buffer.

Substances which are substantive to hair

When amino acids which contain two acid groups and one amino (basic) group join in the formation of a polypeptide chain during keratinisation of the hair in the follicle, one of the acid groups is left free. Similarly amino acids containing two amino groups and one acid group give rise to a free basic group in the hair. If the free acid group of one amino acid lies opposite a free basic group in an adjacent polypeptide chain the two groups will join to form a salt linkage.

However, in hair keratin there are many more amino acids with two acid groups than amino acids with two basic groups, so a large excess of free acid groups is present in the hair (see Fig. 7.2).

Since these acid groups have a negative electrical charge they will attract substances with a positive electrical charge, that is, they attract cations (opposite charges attract each other and like charges repel each other). Such substances, which are attracted to hair and cling to the acid groups electrostatically, are said to be substantive to hair (see Fig. 7.2). They include cationic detergents (quaternary ammonium compounds) such as cetrimide, cationic temporary colours, e.g. methylene blue, polyvinyl pyrrolidone and the amino (basic) group of the amino acids used in 'protein conditioners'. Substantive substances cling to the hair shaft even after the hair has been rinsed and many of the substances are used as conditioners. Cetrimide is useful as an antiseptic as well as a conditioner since the antiseptic properties also persist on the hair after rinsing has been carried out.

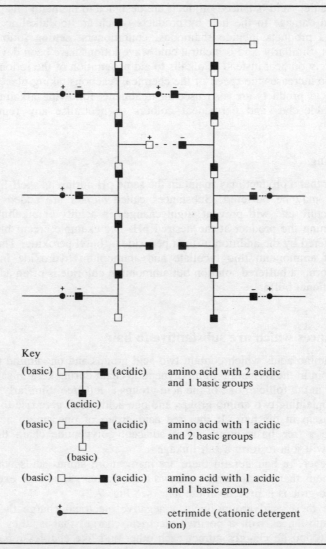

Key

| (basic) □——■ (acidic) | amino acid with 2 acidic and 1 basic groups |
| (acidic) |

(basic) □——■ (acidic)   amino acid with 1 acidic
(basic)   and 2 basic groups

(basic) □——■ (acidic)   amino acid with 1 acidic
                        and 1 basic group

●———   cetrimide (cationic detergent
                        ion)

Fig 7.2 Substances substantive to hair

Protein hydrolysates

Many modern hairdressing preparations, including shampoos, conditioners, pre-bleach and pre-perm 'fillers', perm lotions, bleaches and setting
lotions, contain protein hydrolysates. These consist of mixtures of amino
acids, dipeptides (two amino acids chemically combined) or short
polypeptide chains of amino acids. They are prepared by the *hydrolysis* of

waste animal protein products such as horse hair, feathers, hooves, collagen from hides, or from vegetable proteins such as soya beans.

Hydrolysis is a chemical reaction which involves the decomposition of a substance accompanied by the addition of the elements of water to the substances formed during the decomposition. During the hydrolysis of proteins, polypeptide chains are split into shorter lengths of amino acids or into individual amino acids, water being added as the peptide linkages

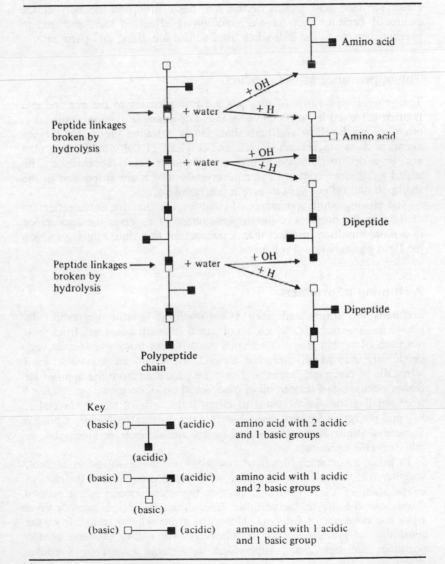

Fig 7.3 Hydrolysis of protein

between the amino acids are broken down (see Fig. 7.3). The reaction is the opposite of the one in which amino acids are joined together to form polypeptide chains during keratinisation. The products of hydrolysis may undergo further treatment including neutralisation by alkalis or triethanolamine. Hydrolysis of the protein materials may be brought about by boiling with hydrochloric acid or by the action of certain enzymes. Some of the molecules of protein hydrolysates are small enough to enter the hairshaft, and are substantive to hair, clinging to either the free acid groups or the free basic group in the polypeptide chains of keratin. They have a conditioning effect on hair, and tend to prevent damage to the hair when used before bleaching and perming.

The appearance of the product

The general appearance of products must be pleasing to the eye and this is often achieved by artificial colouring. For example, lemon shampoo is often coloured yellow and herb shampoo is coloured green. Opacifying agents such as magnesium stearate and ethylene glycol monostearate may also be added to shampoo to give an opaque or pearly appearance. The added substances consist of minute crystals which are suspended in the shampoo and reflect light to give a pearly lustre.

The creamy white appearance of emulsions is also due to the reflection of light by the droplets of the disperse phase. This gives the appearance of a more emollient product than a transparent thin liquid through which the light passes without reflection.

Perfuming of products

Perfumes are formulated from sweet-smelling volatile vegetable oils known as *essential oils*, which are obtained in small quantities from various parts of certain plants. These oils are different from non-volatile vegetable oils such as olive oil and almond oil, which are known as *fixed oils*. Oils of lavender, jasmin and rose are produced from the appropriate flower petals; oil of lemon, oil of orange and oil of bergamot are obtained from small glands in the skins of citrus fruits; oils of thyme, lavender, bay and petitgrain (orange leaves) are obtained from the leaves of plants. Some essential oils are esters, and others are alcohols or aldehydes, or other organic chemicals.

In making perfume, blends of essential oils are dissolved in ethanol, together with certain *animal secretions* which help to equalise the rates of evaporation of the mixed oils so that the same odour is maintained throughout the life of the perfume. The animal secretions include civet from the civet cat of Ethiopia, ambergris from whales, musk from the musk deer of Tibet and castor from beavers. The natural products used in perfumes are now being superseded to a large extent by synthetic materials.

Hairdressing preparations such as lacquers, which are designed to remain on the hair for some time, should be lightly perfumed with highly volatile oils, so that the perfume quickly fades and does not clash with that normally worn by the client. Unpleasant-smelling products such as perm lotions need a strong perfume to mask the odour of the product. The perfuming of perm lotion is often difficult since the reducing agents in the lotion may decompose the ingredients of the perfume.

Product testing by manufacturers

Before marketing new products, exhaustive laboratory and consumer test ing is carried out to ensure the safety of users, to evaluate the performance of the product and to test its stability during storage.

Tests for health hazards

Tests are carried out on proposed new products to ensure there is no danger to the hair itself, the skin, eyes or to the general health of the user. These include tests for primary irritation, and sensitisation tests to avoid, as far as possible, substances which may cause allergic reactions. Patch tests are carried out on the skin of a small number of people and if these prove satisfactory, the tests are extended to include, say, 200 people. A positive reaction even on one person would probably lead to modification or total rejection of the product.

Many chemicals produce serious eye irritation, and tests on shampoos in particular are carried out to avoid the risk of eye damage. Many detergent substances are unsuitable as shampoos for this reason, though in some cases additives to the shampoo will lessen eye irritation. Recent concern about cancer-producing substances has caused an increase in the testing of products, especially of dyes, though such testing is difficult as the effect of cancer-causing materials is not obvious for months or even years afterwards.

Performance tests

The effect of proposed new products is often tested by the *half head test*, in which the product is applied to only half a client's head so that the new product may be compared directly with a standard existing product applied to the other half of the hair. This type of test is used to evaluate the performance of shampoos, conditioners and perm lotions.

Before being marketed, new dyes are used in trials to test colour permanence and fading on exposure to sunlight.

Shelf life tests

Products must be manufactured so that they retain the same qualities throughout normal storage or shelf life. They are tested to guard against possible change of colour in the product, change of pH, perfume deterioration, emulsion breakdown and damage by bacterial or mould growth.

Correct storage conditions in the salon are, of course, essential to avoid deterioration and products should always be stored in a dry place away from direct sunlight and sources of heat.

Experiment 7.4   Half head tests

Compare various shampoos by using one shampoo on the right half of a fellow student's head and a second shampoo on the left half by parting the hair down the mid-line of the scalp.

Compare the result of using a 'protein' shampoo on one side and normal triethanolamine lauryl sulphate shampoo on the other. Also compare a herb shampoo with a lemon shampoo in the same way, noting lustre, feel, etc.

The same type of test can be carried out using a pre-perm filler on one half of the head only, before perming the whole head. Conditioning rinses may also be applied to half the head only, to estimate their effectiveness.

Questions

1. Using a 12 per cent hydrogen peroxide solution and deionised water, describe how you would obtain:
   (a) 20 ml of 9 per cent hydrogen peroxide;   (b) 30 ml of 6 per cent hydrogen peroxide;   (c) 40 ml of 3 per cent hydrogen peroxide.
2. What is meant by the cracking of an emulsion?
   Give an example of a hairdressing product in which it is essential that the emulsion cracks easily, and one where the emulsion must be stable.
3. Estimate the pH value of:
   (a) an acid-balanced shampoo;   (b) a potassium soap shampoo;   (c) a triethanolamine lauryl sulphate shampoo.
4. State one use in hairdressing of:
   (a) ethyl acetate;   (b) carnauba wax;   (c) isopropanol.
5. What are the products of decomposition of hydrogen peroxide?
   What substance is contained in bleaches to cause this decomposition?
6. Explain why many hairdressing products are made alkaline.
   Discuss the effect of various strengths of alkalis on hair. What are the uses of the alkalis, sodium hydroxide and ammonium hydroxide in hairdressing?
7. Describe the structure of an oil-in-water emulsion and explain why an emulsifying agent is necessary to produce a stable emulsion. Give three examples of hairdressing products which are often formulated as emulsions and list the main ingredients in each case.
8. Explain what is meant by:
   (a) an acid-balanced product;   (b) a protein hydrolysate;
   (c) a half head test.

9. Describe the various products used in the manufacture of perfumes and indicate the usefulness of each product.
10. Discuss the use in hairdressing products of:
    (a) silicone fluids;   (b) petroleum products;   (c) vegetable oils.

Chapter 8

Shampoos

Shampoos consist of substances which are designed to assist in the cleansing of hair by the removal of grease, particulate dirt, dead skin scales and various hairdressing preparations such as control creams and lacquers. They must not only clean the hair but also leave it in good condition, soft and smooth to the touch, lustrous and manageable. Such substances include solvents, dry absorbent powders and surface active detergents.

Solvents have a very limited use for cleaning hair except as wig cleaners. White spirit (petroleum liquid) is occasionally used in men's hairdressing and trichloroethane is used as a wig-cleaner. In general however solvents are either highly flammable or highly toxic, and no really satisfactory solvent is available for use on clients. *Dry powders*, which absorb grease when brushed through the hair, are also rarely used in salon work. They usually consist of talc, Fuller's earth, starch or French chalk together with an alkaline substance such as borax or sodium carbonate (washing soda). Most salon shampoos are *surface active detergents*, either soaps or soapless (non-soap) types which are used in conjunction with water.

A large number of the substances classed as detergents are unsuitable as shampoos because they are too alkaline and therefore harsh to the hair, are irritant to the eyes, are not sufficiently soluble in water or do not produce a good lather. Some detergents, such as those used in automatic washing machines, will clean effectively with little or no lather, but the clothes are kept in contact with the detergent by being constantly tumbled through the detergent solution. In shampooing, the lather helps to keep a concentrated solution of detergent in close contact with the hair and skin, enabling the detergent to be moved easily over their surfaces and also acting as a visible guide to the amount of detergent required.

The structure and properties of detergents

Although there are many types of detergents, detergency depends on the presence of both a *hydrophilic* (a water-loving) group and a *hydrophobic* (water-hating) group of atoms either in the detergent molecule itself or in the ions produced in detergent solutions.

The hydrophobic group usually consists of a long hydrocarbon chain (consisting only of carbon and hydrogen atoms) forming a long tail which avoids water. The tail is joined to a hydrophilic 'head' which may carry an electrical charge. The detergent may thus be represented as shown in Fig. 8.1. This structure causes the detergent to form a *mono-layer* (a single layer of molecules) at the junction or interface between air and water (see Fig. 8.2) and between oil (or grease) and water (see Fig. 8.3).

The formation of a similar layer of detergent on the surface of a droplet of water *lowers the surface tension of the water*, and makes the droplet flatten out to 'wet' the surface with which it is in contact (see Fig. 8.4). Thus the detergent acts as a *wetting agent*.

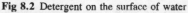

Hydrophobic tail   Hydrophilic head

Fig 8.1 Structure of detergent

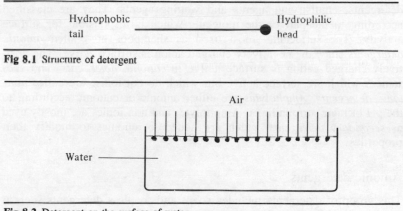

Air

Water

Fig 8.2 Detergent on the surface of water

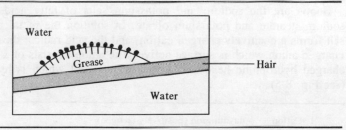

Water

Grease

Hair

Water

Fig 8.3 Detergent at interface between water and grease

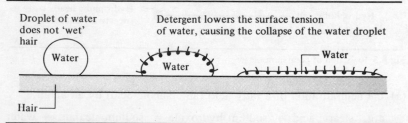

Droplet of water does not 'wet' hair

Detergent lowers the surface tension of water, causing the collapse of the water droplet

Water

Water

Water

Hair

Fig 8.4 Use of detergent to lower surface tension

Detergents also act as *emulsifying agents* by surrounding droplets of oil and holding them suspended in water to form an emulsion. They are also responsible for the formation of foams (lathers).

Due to these properties detergents are said to be 'surface active' and they belong to a group of substances called *surface active agents* or surfactants.

Types of surfactant

Surfactants include a large number of substances which are used as detergents, emulsifying agents and wetting agents. They are classified according to the part of the molecule which is responsible for surface activity. The surfactants most used as shampoos are called *anionic detergents* since the negatively charged anion is surface active. The positively charged cation is surface active in *cationic detergents*, and substances which are surface active but which do not ionise are called *non-ionic detergents*. *Ampholytes* are either anionic or cationic according to the pH of their surroundings. Ampholytes and non-ionics are mostly used as *secondary detergents* which are added to anionics to modify their properties.

Anionic detergents

This group of detergents includes soaps and soapless detergents such as the lauryl sulphates and sulphonated oils. In each case the substances ionise and the anion is surface active.

Soaps are the sodium and potassium salts of fatty acids, such as sodium stearate and potassium oleate. In solution the metal part of the salt forms a positively charged cation, and the acid radical the negatively charged anion which is surface active. The anion consists of a negatively charged hydrophilic head and a hydrocarbon tail which is hydrophobic (see Fig. 8.5).

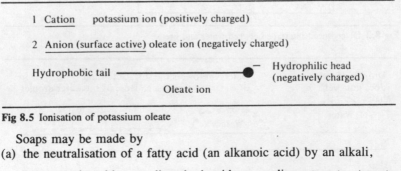

1 <u>Cation</u>   potassium ion (positively charged)

2 <u>Anion (surface active)</u> oleate ion (negatively charged)

Hydrophobic tail ————————————●⁻ Hydrophilic head (negatively charged)

Oleate ion

Fig 8.5 Ionisation of potassium oleate

Soaps may be made by
(a) the neutralisation of a fatty acid (an alkanoic acid) by an alkali,

e.g. stearic acid + sodium hydroxide = sodium stearate + water
(soap)

$$\text{an acid} \quad + \quad \text{an alkali} \quad = \quad \text{a salt} \quad + \text{water}$$

(b) saponification which involves boiling animal fats (beef or mutton fat) or vegetable oils (castor, coconut palm or olive oil) with an alkali,

e.g. olive oil + potassium hydroxide $\xrightarrow{\text{boil}}$ potassium oleate + glycerol

$$\text{vegetable oil} + \quad\quad \text{alkali} \quad\quad \xrightarrow{\text{boil}} \quad\quad \text{soap} \quad\quad + \text{glycerol}$$

Manufacturers produce different types of soap by varying the mixture of oil and fats and also the form of alkali used. *Hard soaps* used as household and toilet soaps and also soap powders, are made by boiling animal fats with sodium hydroxide. *Soft soaps*, which are used in shampoos, are made by boiling vegetable oil with potassium hydroxide or triethanolamine. Glycerol, which is a by-product of soap-making, is removed from hard soaps by a process called 'salting out'. Common salt (sodium chloride) is added when boiling is completed, and since soap is insoluble in salt solution it separates out. The soap floats on top of the salt and glycerol, which may then be drained off from below. In the case of soft soap the glycerol is left in the soap.

Soapless detergents were first produced in the form of sulphonated oils made by treating vegetable oils, especially castor and olive oil, with sulphuric acid. Sulphonated castor oil, known also as Turkey Red oil, and sulphonated olive oil are still used as conditioning shampoos as they act as an oil and a detergent at the same time and are easily rinsed off the hair.

Sulphonated alcohols have for a long time formed the largest group of soapless detergents used as shampoos. They are made by treating lauryl alcohol (dodecanol), obtained from coconut oil or more recently synthesised from petroleum products, with sulphuric acid to form lauryl hydrogen sulphate. Neutralisation of the lauryl hydrogen sulphate by various alkalis gives a variety of products used as shampoos (see Table 8.1).

Table 8.1 Preparation of soapless detergents

	Alkali		Detergent	Properties of detergent
Lauryl hydrogen sulphate	+	Sodium hydroxide	→ Sodium lauryl sulphate	A white paste used in cream shampoos. Not very soluble in water so unsuitable for clear shampoo. Tends to be harsh on hair
Lauryl hydrogen sulphate	+	Ammonium hydroxide	→ Ammonium lauryl sulphate	A thick amber liquid
Lauryl hydrogen sulphate	+	Triethanol-amine	→ Triethanol amine lauryl sulphate (TLS)	A thin colourless liquid with good foaming properties. Used in clear liquid shampoos. Mild to hair
Lauryl hydrogen sulphate	+	Monoethanol-amine	→ Monoethanol-amine lauryl sulphate	Thicker than TLS, so easier to apply. Mild to hair

Ionisation of the lauryl sulphate detergents gives rise to a surface active anion with a negatively charged hydrophilic head and a hydrocarbon tail which is hydrophobic (see Fig. 8.6).

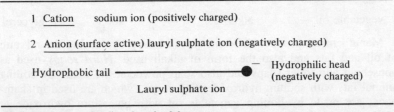

1 Cation   sodium ion (positively charged)

2 Anion (surface active) lauryl sulphate ion (negatively charged)

Hydrophobic tail ⎯⎯⎯⎯⎯⎯⎯⎯⎯● ⁻ Hydrophilic head (negatively charged)

Lauryl sulphate ion

Fig 8.6 Ionisation of sodium lauryl sulphate

More modern types of soapless detergents used as shampoos include: **Sodium lauryl ether sulphate** made by treating lauryl alcohol with ethylene oxide to form an ether, before sulphating with sulphuric acid and neutralising with sodium hydroxide. Sodium lauryl ether sulphate is milder on the hair, less degreasing and more soluble than sodium lauryl sulphate. It forms a clear liquid shampoo, the viscosity of which may be adjusted by use of sodium chloride (common salt) and it can therefore be used in very thick clear products.
Sodium lauryl sarcosinate is often used in aerosol shampoos as it has a very much lower corrosive effect on the metal of aerosol cans than other soapless detergents.

Cationic detergents

The most important group of cationic detergents used in hairdressing belong to a class of salts known as *quaternary ammonium salts* (quats). These include such substances as cetyl trimethyl ammonium bromide (cetrimide), distearyl dimethyl ammonium chloride and alkyl dimethyl benzyl ammonium chloride (ADBAC). They ionise to give a surface active cation (see Fig. 8.7).

The most commonly used of these compounds in hairdressing products is cetrimide. Pure cetrimide is a white powder which is soluble in both water and alcohol. Since it does not produce a good lather it is not used

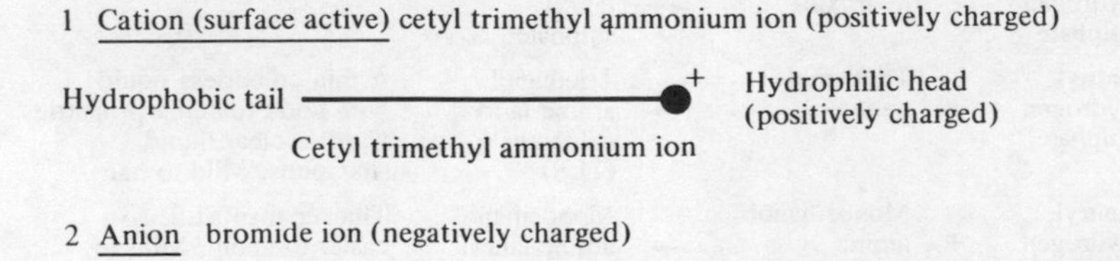

1 Cation (surface active) cetyl trimethyl ammonium ion (positively charged)

Hydrophobic tail ⎯⎯⎯⎯⎯⎯⎯⎯⎯● ⁺ Hydrophilic head (positively charged)

Cetyl trimethyl ammonium ion

2 Anion   bromide ion (negatively charged)

Fig 8.7 Ionisation of cetrimide

as a regular shampoo, but it has antiseptic properties which make it suitable for occasional use as a medicated shampoo. Cetrimide is substantive to hair due to the positive charge on its surface active cation, so it clings electrostatically to the acid groups in hair keratin and its effect persists even after rinsing. More cetrimide is taken up by damaged hair due to an increase in the number of free acid groups when hair is damaged. It leaves hair soft and smooth, so adds lustre and reduces the possibility of fly-away hair.

The antiseptic properties of cetrimide make it useful:

(a) as a medicated shampoo;
(b) for the immersion of tools in the antiseptic bowl used on dressing out tables;
(c) in barrier creams.

The conditioning properties of cetrimide make it useful in:

(a) cream rinses used after shampooing, perming, bleaching and colouring;
(b) perm lotions;
(c) neutralisers.

The main disadvantages of cetrimide are:

(a) Its poor lather makes it unsuitable for regular shampoos.
(b) In concentrations above 2 per cent, cetrimide products may cause permanent opacity of the cornea of the eye (the transparent tissue in front of the lens of the eye).
(c) It may act, in some people, as a sensitiser producing later allergic reaction.
(d) It is incompatible with anionic detergents. Cetrimide cannot be mixed with soap or lauryl sulphates as the oppositely charged surface active ions destroy the detergent properties of both. Anionic shampoos must therefore be washed thoroughly from the hair before applying a cetrimide rinse.

Ampholytes

These detergents are anionic in alkaline solutions and cationic in acid solutions. They do not foam well, so are not used alone as shampoos but 2–3 per cent is often added to anionic shampoos as a *secondary detergent*. The most commonly used ampholyte is lauryl betaine.

When added to soaps and lauryl sulphate shampoos, ampholytes

(a) stabilise the foam, preventing premature foam-collapse;
(b) increase the amount of lather;
(c) make anionics less irritant to the eyes;
(d) increase the viscosity of the shampoo;
(e) act as conditioners, since they are substantive to hair;
(f) add weak antiseptic properties to the shampoo.

Ampholytes such as coconut imidazoline are now being added in larger quantities (up to 20 per cent) to anionic detergents, to produce very mild shampoos.

Non-ionic detergents

Substances which do not ionise, but which have surface-active molecules, are known as non-ionic detergents. The main ones used in hairdressing products are *alkanolamides* (alkylolamides), usually lauryl monoethanolamide (sometimes called coconut monoethanolamide), and lauryl diethanolamide (coconut diethanolamide). These are waxy solids which are insoluble in water but soluble in anionic detergents. They produce little foam themselves but are compatible with anionics, and when 3–5 per cent is added to a soapless shampoo it has a foam-boosting effect and increases the viscosity of the shampoo. Alkanolamides are substantive to hair so have a conditioning effect also. The addition of 2 per cent lauryl diethanolamide enables a clear shampoo to be made from sodium lauryl sulphate, since the alkanolamide increases the solubility of sodium lauryl sulphate. Alkanolamides are also added to soap shampoo since they prevent the formation of a scum of lime soap in hard water.

Lauryl diethanolamide is also used as

(a) a gelling agent in bleaches;
(b) an antistatic in lacquers;
(c) a wetting agent in cold wave lotions;
(d) an emulsifying agent in creams and lotions.

Detergent action during shampooing

The purpose of shampooing is primarily to clean hair by removal of grease and with it dirt and dead scales from the scalp, though it may be used to assist in carrying out other hairdressing processes. Removal of grease before perming assists the entry of perm lotion into the cortex; whilst shampooing before setting enables water to enter the cortex more easily so increasing elasticity and producing a better set. Water alone will

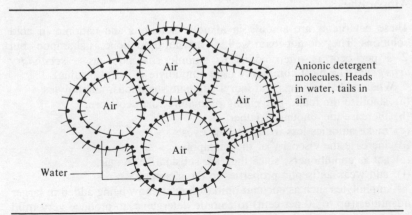

Anionic detergent molecules. Heads in water, tails in air

Fig 8.8 Foam structure

not clean hair as it will not mix with grease, and due to its surface tension does not easily 'wet' surfaces. The addition of detergent overcomes these difficulties, and a detergent may be defined as 'a substance used with water for cleansing purposes'.

When the shampoo is applied to the wet hair the detergent lowers the surface tension of the water, and layers of detergent solution trap pockets of air to create *a foam* when the scalp is massaged. The detergent forms a mono-layer between the water and air in much the same way as it forms a layer between oil and water in an emulsion, (see Fig. 8.8). In fact, a foam is similar to an emulsion, the disperse phase being a gas (air) and the continuous phase, water.

Since the shampoo is an anionic detergent, the hydrophilic heads of the detergent ion enter the water and the hydrophobic tails stay in the air of the bubble, so forming a bridge between the air and the water. The negative charges on the 'heads' repel each other, tending to make the bubble thicker and therefore more stable. If the liquid film is thick the bubbles are spherical, but if the film is thin the bubbles form a figure with twelve flat sides (a dodecahedron), each side being a regular pentagon (five

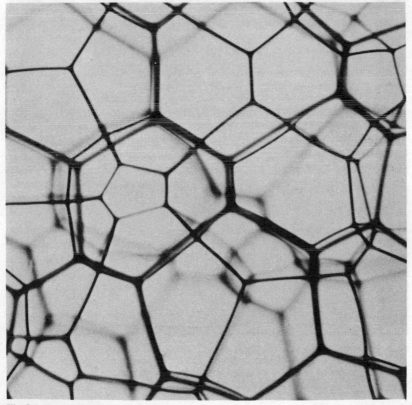

Fig 8.9 Foam structure

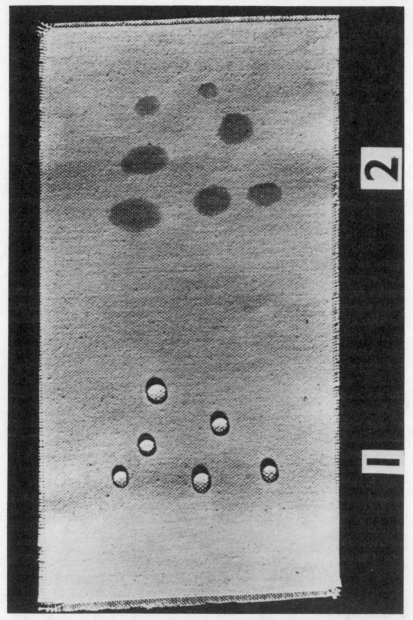

Fig 8.10 Detergent acts as a wetting agent. (1) Globules of ordinary tap water on the surface of unbleached cotton fabric. (2) Water mixed with detergent (Teepol) – increased surface wetting and also deep penetration of the fabric's structure

sides) (see Fig. 8.9). The sides of each bubble are shared with adjacent bubbles. Small spherical bubbles give a more stable foam and shampoos are formulated to give this type of bubble. The massaging of the shampoo into the hair and scalp helps to dislodge loose scale and dirt.

The detergent also acts as a wetting agent, that is, it lowers the surface tension of water to bring the water into closer contact with the hair (see Fig. 8.10). It must not however wet the hair too much, or it will be difficult to dry out. Hair may absorb up to about 30 per cent of its own weight of water, and about two thirds of this will have to be evaporated off during drying to give the normal water content of about 10 per cent.

During shampooing, the hydrophobic tails of the anions enter the grease whilst the hydrophilic heads stay in the water (see Fig. 8.11a, b, c). The negative charges on the heads of the ions repel each other, causing the grease to 'roll up' (see Fig. 8.12), become dislodged from the hair and form an oil-in-water emulsion (see Fig. 8.11). The detergent thus acts as an emulsifying agent.

Hot water used in shampooing helps to make the grease more mobile and an emulsion is formed more easily because of the higher temperature. The mechanical removal of grease from the hair also takes place by massage. Solid particles of dirt (particulate dirt) are usually attached to the grease and the two are removed together.

The droplets of grease in the emulsion repel each other due to the negative charge on the ions surrounding the grease, so the droplets are prevented from joining to form larger droplets which could be redeposited on the hair. The detergent also forms a layer on the surface of the hair with the tails next to the hair and the heads in the water. Thus there is also a force of repulsion between the oil droplets and the hair (see Fig. 8.11). The grease is not redeposited on the hair but is held

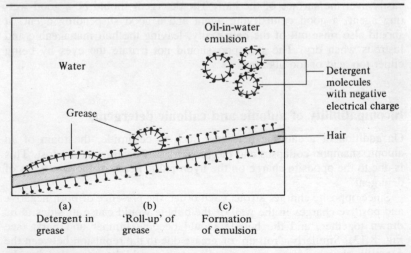

(a) Detergent in grease
(b) 'Roll-up' of grease
(c) Formation of emulsion

Fig 8.11(a)(b)(c) Detergent action

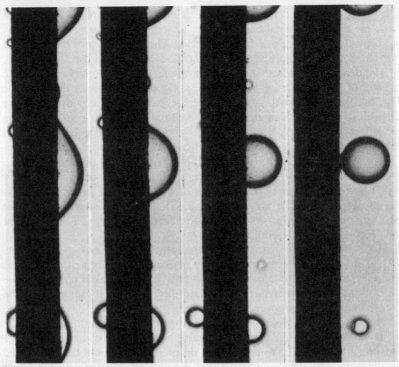

Fig 8.12 Detergent action to show 'roll-up' of grease

suspended in the water until it is rinsed away, so the detergent acts as a suspending agent.

A good shampoo should therefore form a creamy lather which spreads easily over the surface of the hair. The detergent should be a good wetting agent, a good emulsifying agent and a good suspending agent. It should also rinse out of the hair easily, leaving the hair manageable and lustrous when dry. The shampoo should not irritate the eyes by being either too acid or too alkaline.

Incompatibility of anionic and cationic detergents

On addition of a cationic detergent such as cetrimide, the foam of an anionic shampoo collapses and the properties of detergency are lost. This is due to the opposite charge on the hydrophilic heads of the two types of detergent.

Since opposite charges attract each other, the presence of both negative and positive charges in the wall of the bubble would cause its sides to be drawn together, and the bubble would become thinner and burst (see Fig. 8.13). Similarly, 'roll up' of grease due to the repulsion between the negative charges of the anionic detergent would be cancelled by the

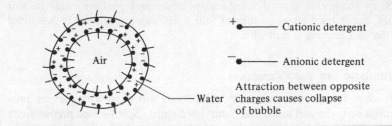

Fig 8.13 Foam collapse by mixing anionic and cationic detergents

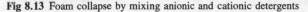

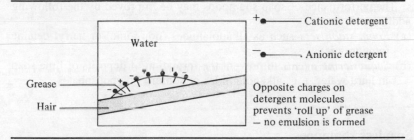

Fig 8.14 Prevention of roll-up

positive charges of the cationic detergent and an emulsion would not be formed (see Fig. 8.14).

In some cases the mixing of solutions of anionic and cationic detergents results in the formation of complex insoluble salts, so these are precipitated from the solution and detergent effect is lost in this way. Thus anionic and cationic detergents cannot be used in the same products and anionic shampoos must be well rinsed from the hair before applying cationic conditioning rinses.

Soap shampoos

Potassium palmitate and potassium oleate, the soft soaps traditionally used as shampoos, are always alkaline with a pH of 8–9, so are harsh to the hair, leaving it rough and dull. The few soap shampoos now available contain triethanolamine oleate or monoethanolamine oleate, which are less alkaline with a pH of 7.5–8 and are therefore milder. Super fatted soaps (olive oil soaps) are also less alkaline. The olive oil added during manufacture contains oleic acid which neutralises the normal alkalinity of the soap.

Soaps are precipitated by acids so it is impossible to form an acid-based soap shampoo. They are also insoluble in salt solutions (sodium chloride solution) so soap will not lather in salt water. When washing sea water from the hair, the salt should be well rinsed away with clean water before attempting to use soap.

Soap shampoos give a satisfactory lather and perform well in soft water, but in hard water a scum of lime soap (calcium oleate) is deposited on the hair leaving a dull film.

Formulation of soap shampoo

Soft soap shampoos are made by dilution of soft soap with varying proportions of water and industrial methylated spirit. Spirit-based preparations are useful as lacquer–removing shampoos for shellac-based lacquers. Shellac is insoluble in water but soluble in alcohol.

The performance of soap shampoos may be improved by the following additives:

(a) *Foam stabilisers* such as alkanolamides (non-ionic) or lauryl betaine (ampholytic).
(b) *Sequestering agents* to prevent the formation of deposits of lime soap in hard water, e.g. alkanolamides or sodium polyphosphates.

Soapless shampoos

The soapless detergents such as triethanolamine lauryl sulphate and sodium lauryl sulphate are usually neutral or slightly alkaline (pH 7–7.5) so are generally milder to the hair than soap shampoos. Since they are unaffected by acids, most soapless detergents are now formulated to give a pH of 6.5 to 7 by the addition of citric acid. Acid balanced shampoos with a pH of 4.5–5.5 are also possible. Soapless detergents do not form a scum with the salts in hard water, and can be used to wash salt water from the hair. Their main disadvantages are that they tend to degrease the hair too much and often cause dermatitis.

The formulation of soapless shampoos

Soapless detergents form the basis of a wide variety of types of shampoos.

Clear liquid shampoos may contain 10–20 per cent of mono-ethanolamine lauryl sulphate, triethanolamine lauryl sulphate or sodium lauryl ether sulphate. They may be thickened by the addition of sodium chloride, ammonium chloride or sodium alginate. Foam boosters such as alkanolamides and lauryl betaine may be added and these also act as conditioners. Polyvinyl pyrrolidone may also be added as a conditioner and to reduce eye irritation.

Liquid cream shampoos are similar to clear liquid shampoos, but are made opaque by the addition of a soap such as magnesium stearate, which gives a pearly appearance. Foam boosters may be added as for clear liquid shampoos.

Solid cream shampoos contain 25 per cent sodium lauryl sulphate thickened by the addition of small quantities of soap. Lanolin may be added as a conditioner.

Gel shampoos contain 20–25 per cent of triethanolamine lauryl sulphate thickened by methyl cellulose, alkanolamide or by synthetic gums.

Powder shampoos are not popular as they have to be dissolved in warm water before use. They contain spray-dried sodium lauryl sulphate.

Aerosol shampoos are dispensed as a foam which is formed as the product leaves the can. The aerosol propellent vaporises and the gas, expanding as it leaves the can passes into the detergent solution, forming bubbles. Mixtures of sodium lauryl sulphate and triethanolamine lauryl sulphate may be used, but as these corrode metals the aerosol container is often glass though this may be plastic covered. Sodium lauryl sarcosinate is now frequently used since it is less corrosive, and a metal container is satisfactory.

Modification of soapless shampoos for special purposes

In addition to shampoos intended for hair in normally good condition, shampoos may be adapted for special purposes.

For greasy hair the percentage of soapless detergent in the shampoo may be increased from the normal 15–20 per cent up to 50 per cent. Lemon and lime shampoos are often associated with shampoos for greasy hair but there is no advantage in such shampoos.

For dry hair several alternatives are available:
(a) The percentage of soapless detergent may be as low as 10 per cent to make the shampoo less 'de-greasing'.
(b) Oils such as olive oil, coconut oil and almond oil may be added to the shampoo to increase the amount of oil on the hair.
(c) A sulphonated oil shampoo may be used as this acts as an oil and a detergent at the same time.
(d) The amount of lanolin in the shampoo may be increased.
(e) Other conditioners such as beer, egg and herbs may be added but have little value since they are quickly rinsed from the hair. Beer is better applied as a final rinse when it stiffens the hair slightly. Some herbs have a slight antiseptic quality but are mostly used for their perfume.

Medicated shampoos are of two types both of which are based on antiseptics. They have a limited effect on dandruff since they do not reduce scaling, but will reduce the number of micro-organisms on the scalp.
(a) *Cationic detergent shampoos* (cetrimide shampoos) are useful since cetrimide is substantive to hair and the antiseptic film remains even after rinsing. This type of shampoo does not give a good lather but is easily rinsed from the hair. These shampoos are best applied using a backwash basin as cetrimide is damaging to the eyes.
(b) *Soapless shampoos with added antiseptics*. These shampoos are most satisfactory if the antiseptic is substantive to hair, otherwise the effect

is lost on rinsing. The most frequently used antiseptics are trichlorocarbanalide and hexachlorophane, but bithionol, coal tar and resorcinol are possible.

Antidandruff shampoos contain substances which inhibit the multiplication of the cells of the stratum germinativium in the epidermis. Zinc pyrithione (zinc omadine) is a good antiseptic as well as preventing multiplication of cells, and about 2–3 per cent is usually used in a lauryl ether sulphate detergent base. Selenium sulphide (2–5 per cent) in a soapless detergent base is also used but sometimes gives rise to dermatitis.

Brightening shampoos are used to give highlights to light brown hair or to revive blonde hair which has darkened with age. The most effective contain 3 per cent hydrogen peroxide added to a soapless shampoo. Camomile, a vegetable dye obtained by infusion of dried camomile flowers, is sometimes added to shampoo bases as a brightener but its effect is slight.

Colour shampoos may be formulated by the addition of temporary dyes (azo-dyes), semi-permanent dyes or vegetable dyes to a soapless shampoo base. The use of vegetable dyes has increased recently and both henna, used to give red highlights to black hair, and walnut, used to revive the colour of dark brown hair, are available.

Protein shampoos do not contain protein itself but the products of the breakdown of protein by hydrolysis. The shampoos thus contain mixtures of amino acids, dipeptides or short chains of amino acids in a shampoo base. The protein hydrolysates are substantive to hair and so have a conditioning effect, making the hair smoother and adding lustre. Many of the amino acids will cling to the outside of the hair shaft, but on damaged hair, which is more porous, some will enter the cortex. 'Split ends' may be made to cling together but there is no permanent repair.

Acid-balanced shampoos are designed to keep the hair in its natural acid state, or to return the hair to that state after alkaline treatments such as bleaching, tinting and perming. The swelling of the hair caused by alkalis is reduced, the cuticle is left well aligned and its surface smooth. Acid-balanced shampoos help to stop the fading of tinted hair by keeping the cuticle scales closed during shampooing. They are mostly based on ammonium lauryl sulphate detergents as these are particularly stable in acid conditions. The pH is usually adjusted to 4.5–5.5.

Questions

1. How do soap shampoos react with:
   (a) acids;   (b) hard water;   (c) solutions of common salt?
2. What is meant by:
   (a) saponification;   (b) a superfatted soap;   (c) a sulphonated oil.

3. Explain why nonionic detergents and ampholytes are termed 'secondary detergents'.

4. Name (a) a solvent used in wig cleaning;   (b) a substance which is a by-product of soap making;   (c) a cationic detergent.

5. Describe the structure of a detergent molecule.

6. What are the properties of a good shampoo?
   Discuss the advantages and disadvantages of the use of soapless shampoos in preference to soap-based shampoos.

7. Discuss the importance of a lather in shampooing. Describe the structure of a foam and name the substances added to shampoos to help to stabilise the lather. What is the effect of a cationic detergent on the lather of a soapless shampoo?

8. With the aid of diagrams explain how a soapless detergent shampoo assists in the process of cleaning hair during shampooing.

9. Explain how a soapless detergent shampoo may be modified for use as:

   (a) a medicated shampoo;   (b) a conditioning shampoo;
   (c) an anti-dandruff shampoo;   (d) a brightening shampoo;
   (e) a shampoo for greasy hair.

10. What is meant by a detergent? Discuss the various types of detergent available and describe their uses in hairdressing products.

Chapter 9

Changing the colour of hair

The natural colour of hair is an inherited characteristic due mainly to the presence of pigment granules which are deposited in the cortex of the hair during its development in the follicle. The natural colour may be made lighter by bleaching, or extra colour may be added to the natural colour during the process of dyeing. In some cases the two processes may be carried out together, and the hair may be dyed lighter than the natural shade.

Natural hair colour

During the development of hair follicles in the foetus, melanocytes, which are colour-producing and distributing cells, are carried down from the germinating layer of the epidermis to lie amongst the cells surrounding the upper part of the papilla. Melanin in the form of granules is produced by these cells, and transferred to the passing cortical cells by means of the dendrites of the active melanocytes.

Actual hair colour depends mainly on:
1. The amount of pigment produced by the melanocytes (not on the number of melanocytes, as some may be inactive).
2. The colour of the pigment. This may be:
   (a) a black or brown pigment known as melanin;
   (b) a red or yellow pigment known as pheomelanin;
   (c) a red pigment known as trichosiderin (a complex iron compound).

Mixtures of these differently coloured pigments give rise to various shades of hair (see Table 9.1).

Table 9.1 Hair colour

Colour of hair	Combination of pigments
Blonde	Red and yellow
Light brown	Red, yellow and brown
Dark brown	Red, brown and black
Black	Large amount of black
White	No pigment

To a minor extent the colour is affected by:
1. The reflection of light by the cuticle scales and by the air spaces in the cortex, which gives highlights to hair.

2. A pale yellow colouring matter distributed throughout the cortical fibres, and called fluid pigment or diffused pigment.

Lack of colour in hair

Failure of melanocytes to produce pigment results in white hair. A grey head of hair is considered to be due to a mixture of white and coloured hairs. Melanin is formed in the melanocytes by the oxidation of the amino acid tyrosine, the reaction being brought about by the enzyme tyrosinase (a compound of protein with copper). Thus lack of hair colour may be due to:

1. Lack of tyrosine (caused by shortage of protein in the diet).
2. Lack of copper in the diet, though this is rare as only minute traces of copper are required.
3. Failure by the body to produce the enzyme tyrosinase.

Lack of protein in the diet is rare in this country but in some developing countries small children sometimes suffer from protein deficiency with consequent loss of hair colour. Failure by the body to produce the enzyme tyrosinase is thought to be the cause of loss of colour through ageing. Genetic failure to produce the enzyme results in albinism in which there is lack of colour in the hair, eyes and skin.

Bleaching

During bleaching, melanin and pheomelanin in the hair cortex are oxidised to colourless compounds.

$$\text{melanin} \quad + \quad \text{oxygen} \quad = \quad \text{oxy-melanin}$$
$$\text{(black or brown)} \qquad\qquad\qquad \text{(colourless)}$$

The aim in bleaching is to oxidise the melanin with as little oxidation of disulphide linkages as possible, to minimise hair damage. Bleaches consist basically of two parts:

An oxidising agent, usually hydrogen peroxide but occasionally magnesium peroxide, to provide the oxygen for bleaching.

An alkaline substance, usually ammonium hydroxide solution or solid ammonium carbonate, to act as a catalyst in breaking down the hydrogen peroxide to release oxygen. This part of the bleaching preparation is often thickened, forming a paste bleach, an oil bleach or a cream bleach. These are mixed with hydrogen peroxide immediately before use.

The rate of bleaching may be speeded up by heat from a steamer or infra-red heater.

The oxidising agent

Hydrogen peroxide readily decomposes into water and oxygen when made slightly alkaline.

$$\text{hydrogen peroxide} \longrightarrow \text{water} + \text{nascent oxygen}$$

The newly formed oxygen is known as *nascent oxygen* and is more powerful as a bleach than atmospheric oxygen. Nascent oxygen consists of single atoms of oxygen, and if there is no suitable oxidisable substance available at the time of their formation, they combine in pairs to form oxygen molecules such as those normally present in air.

The amount of oxygen produced and hence the degree of bleaching, depends on the strength of peroxide used. The volume strength and percentage strength of hydrogen peroxide has been discussed in Chapter 7.

Three per cent (10 volume) hydrogen peroxide is used in brightening shampoos, and 6 per cent – 9 per cent (20–30 volume) in normal bleaching. At concentrations higher than 9 per cent hydrogen peroxide will burn the skin, but 9–12 per cent (30–40 vol) may be used for tipping, frosting or bleached streaks, since in these cases the hydrogen peroxide does not come into direct contact with the skin.

The alkali

Small quantities of ammonium hydroxide are used in bleaching to act as a catalyst in the release of oxygen from hydrogen peroxide. The alkali also acts as a wetting agent, causing swelling of the hair and allowing easy entry of the bleach into the cortex. It also neutralises the acid stabiliser (salicylic or phosphoric acid) which is added to hydrogen peroxide during manufacture to prevent premature loss of oxygen.

Types of bleach.

Simple liquid bleaches

Six per cent hydrogen peroxide solution with a small quantity of 0.88 ammonium hydroxide may be used in shampoo as a simple liquid bleach, the shampoo helping to hold the bleach in contact with the hair. The method is rarely used, as cream, oil and paste bleaches are more satisfactory.

Cream bleaches

A cream bleach consists of an alkaline cream (an emulsion) incorporating sequestering agents such as polyphosphates which remove any traces of copper and iron salts on the hair. If allowed to remain, these salts could cause hair damage by producing vigorous catalytic breakdown of the hydrogen peroxide. Buffers of urea peroxide or butyl peroxide are added to keep the pH constant at about 9. The cream is mixed with 6 per cent (20 vol) hydrogen peroxide immediately before use.

Oil bleaches

Some oil bleaches contain sulphonated castor oil (Turkey Red oil) as a thickener, but most are now based on the use of gelling agents. An oil bleach thus consists of a mixture of:

An alkali, usually ammonium hydroxide, to give a pH of 9–9.5. This makes the hair swell and releases oxygen from the hydrogen peroxide.

A wetting agent, e.g. a cationic detergent.
The gelling agent (thickener), usually a nonionic detergent such as lauryl diethanolamide.
Immediately before use 6 per cent (20 vol) hydrogen peroxide is added and this causes the gelling agent to become more viscous. To increase the efficiency of the bleach, that is to increase the amount of available oxygen, *boosters* may be added. These contain mixtures of potassium persulphate and ammonium persulphate (peroxy salts) which give off extra oxygen. The gelling agent is sometimes added to the booster instead of to the 'oil'. Carbopol (a carboxyl vinyl polymer) is used for this purpose as it gels on contact with the alkali.

Oil bleaches based on sulphonated oils give a golden blonde shade and do not bleach as completely as cream bleaches or paste bleaches. Modern 'oil' bleaches are more efficient and also leave the hair in good condition.

Paste or powder bleaches
Powder bleaches consist of a mixture of two white powders, magnesium carbonate (also known as *white henna*) which forms the bulk of the powder, and ammonium carbonate – used instead of liquid ammonium hydroxide – to release the oxygen from the hydrogen peroxide. Immediately before use the powders are mixed to a paste with 6–9 per cent hydrogen peroxide for general bleaching; or with 9–12 per cent hydrogen peroxide for bleached streaks or tips. Since the hydrogen peroxide is not diluted by any other liquids, paste bleaches are more likely to cause hair damage than cream or oil bleaches and the hair may be left in a rough and porous condition.

Hair damage during bleaching

Damage during bleaching is limited to the hair shaft itself, the hair in the follicle being unaffected. The risk of damage depends largely on the amount of lightening required. Changing dark hair to blonde involves a greater risk than changing light brown hair to blonde or dark hair to light brown. Regrowth tends to be more conspicuous if there is a marked colour change and retouch bleaching is then carried out more frequently, again leading to possible damage. In general, bleaching is much more likely to cause hair damage than tinting or perming. The risk of damage may be lessened by use of 'protein fillers' either before bleaching or in the bleach preparation itself. The amino acids and dipeptides in the 'filler' are substantive to hair and cling electrostatically to both acid and basic groups in the hair, and their presence lessens damage to the linkages in keratin.

The chief dangers in bleaching are as follows:
1. Many disulphide linkages between the polypeptide chains in keratin are oxidised by hydrogen peroxide to form cysteic acid. This means that these linkages are permanently lost and the tensile strength of the hair reduced. Since the number of linkages holding the polypeptide

chains together is considerably smaller, water entering the narrow spaces between the chains by capillary rise may force the chains apart, causing swelling of the hair whenever the hair is wet. When dry, the damaged hair may be straw-like, but when wet it may become soft and water logged and be difficult to dry out. Some oxidation products of keratin are soluble and may be lost from the hair, adding further to the weakening of the hair. Loss of disulphide linkages during bleaching may reduce the possibility of a successful perm if this is later required.

2. The polypeptide chains may themselves be broken by over-oxidation leading to breakage of the hair shaft. This may be the result of either over-processing or the use of concentrated hydrogen peroxide.

3. The hair may be softened and destroyed if the bleach is too alkaline. The maximum pH should be 9.5.

4. Scalp burns may occur if hydrogen peroxide of over 9 per cent (30 vol) strength is allowed on the skin.

5. The cuticle scales may be roughened or destroyed, especially during retouching, if overlapping occurs. The hair may feel harsh and straw-like, and be left extremely porous. Flakes of the cuticle may break off.

Treatment when bleaching is completed

Bleaches must always be washed gently from the hair as soon as the desired stage of bleaching has been reached. Further oxidation can then be prevented by addition of an *antioxidant* (reducing agent) rinse which stops the action of the hydrogen peroxide inside the hair shaft. Ascorbic acid is often used in such rinses since in addition to its properties as a reducing agent, the acid neutralises any excess alkali. It thus returns the hair to its normal acid state, reduces any swelling that has taken place and closes the cuticle scales, making the hair smoother. Acids also precipitate the soluble oxidation products formed in the hair during bleaching, and so prevent their loss. Conditioners of the cetrimide type are also added to the rinse to help to repair any damage to the hair. Damaged hair takes up more cetrimide than undamaged hair, since hair contains a greater number of free acid groups after hair damage. The increased porosity of the hair also enables more cetrimide to enter the cortex. (Ascorbic acid is also known as vitamin C but is not used as a vitamin in this instance.)

Causes of the yellowing of bleached hair

Various substances when applied to bleached hair will tend to cause yellowing. These include

1. Alkaline substances such as soap shampoos.

2. Olive oil, which may be used in hair conditioning treatments. Oxidation of the oil on the hair results in yellowing.

3. Hair lotions containing resorcinol.

Smoking causes discolouration of the frontal hair and frequent exposure to strong sunlight may also cause yellowing due to the action of ultra-violet rays.

Bleach toners

Bleaching may leave the hair with a yellow or reddish tinge and 'toners' are designed to overcome this residual coloration. Temporary colours such as methyl violet or methylene blue may be used in weak solution to disguise the yellowness, e.g. a 'platinum blonde' is obtained by rinsing a bleached head with a 1 in 100 000 methylene blue solution. If too much blue is used the hair may become green (blue + yellow = green).

Most modern 'toners' are specially formulated semi-permanent nitro-dyes. These are designed to give delicate pastel shades, to tone down brassy effects after bleaching, and most toners have a slight violet content to counteract yellowness. Some toners involve a light application of permanent oxidation dyes, and a skin test is required. The use of cream bleaches and some oil bleaches makes toning difficult as the oil prevents the dye from entering the hair shaft.

Adding colour to hair

Natural colour granules of melanin lie in the cortex of the hair, and any added colour looks more natural if it too enters the hair shaft. The ability of colouring material to enter the cortex depends on the size of the colour molecules and the porosity of the hair. Colours with large molecules coat

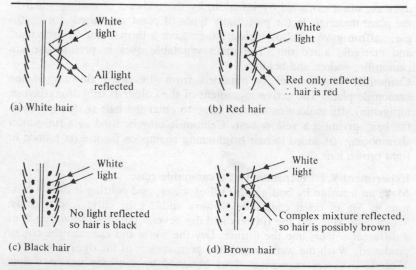

(a) White hair — White light — All light reflected

(b) Red hair — White light — Red only reflected ∴ hair is red

(c) Black hair — White light — No light reflected so hair is black

(d) Brown hair — White light — Complex mixture reflected, so hair is possibly brown

Fig 9.1(a)(b)(c)(d) The colour of hair

the outer surface of the hair only and tend to look dull unless the coating is very fine.

Melanin and the dyes applied to hair produce colour because they contain groupings of atoms called chromophores which have the power to absorb certain wavelengths of light (or colours) from the white daylight or artificial light falling on them; and to reflect others to our eyes. The light which is reflected produces the colour we 'see' and the pigment is named by the reflected colour. Thus we say a pigment is red if it reflects red light and absorbs all other colours. If the pigment of hair absorbs all wavelengths of light and reflects none, the hair appears black (see Fig. 9.1 *a, b, c, d*). If all wavelengths are reflected and none absorbed, the hair appears white. Brown hair reflects a complex mixture of spectrum colours including some red, yellow and blue light.

Types of dye

Hair dyes may be classified in the following groups:
1. Vegetable dyes.
2. Inorganic dyes or metallic dyes.
3. Synthetic organic dyes which may be subdivided into:
    (a) temporary dyes, both anionic and cationic;
    (b) semipermanent dyes or nitro dyes;
    (c) permanent oxidation dyes or para dyes.

Vegetable dyes

Vegetable dyes are obtained from the flowers or leaves of plants. The dyes are often extracted by infusion, by the addition of boiling water to the plant material. In the past many types of plant were used; for example, saffron gave a yellow colour, sage gave a brown tone to grey hair, and marigold a red tint. The main vegetable dyes in present use are camomile, walnut and henna.

Camomile (chamomile) is obtained from the dried flowers of the camomile plant. The active ingredient of the colour is trihydroxyflavone (*apigenin*). Its molecules are too large to enter the hair shaft so it coats the hair, giving it a yellow cast. Camomile may be used as a rinse after shampooing, or added to hair brightening shampoos for use on blonde or light brown hair.

Experiment 9.1   Preparation of a camomile rinse
Make an infusion by boiling 250 ml of water, and pouring it onto a mixture of 5 g of dried camomile flowers and 2 g of citric acid crystals. When cool, filter off the flowers and dip several bundles of hair, each of a different colour, into the filtrate. Dry the wefts and examine the colour produced. Wash the wefts to test the permanence of the dye.

Walnut dyes are permanent dyes obtained by crushing unripe walnut shells. The dye produces a brown colour. Some modern colour shampoos contain walnut juice to deepen the colour of dark brown hair.

Henna is prepared by heating the powdered dried leaves of the Egyptian privet (Lawsonia alba) with water to form a paste. When applied to the hair the paste produces red shades, the exact colour depending on the type of leaf. Leaves collected before maturing produce 'green' henna which gives a more delicate shade. The active ingredient is *lawsone*. The dye molecules are small enough to enter the hair shaft and are oxidised slowly by atmospheric oxygen so that the final permanent colour is not reached for 1–2 days. For this reason the dye is known as a *progressive dye*. It has the advantages of being non-toxic and is unlikely to cause dermatitis.

Henna is used in some modern colour shampoos to give auburn highlights to brown and chestnut hair. Used on black hair it produces red highlights which are particularly noticeable in bright sunlight. When used by itself the range of colour produced by henna is limited to red shades, but these may be modified by the addition of various other substances.

1. The addition of an alkaline substance such as borax makes henna browner.
2. The addition of an acid, e.g. acetic acid, makes henna redder.
3. Used with metallic salts (copper or silver salts) and pyrogallol, black and brown colours are produced, the mixture being known as compound henna or henna rastick.
4. Used with other vegetable dyes such as walnut or indigo, henna becomes modified to form black and brown colours. At one time indigo was obtained from the plant of that name grown in the Middle East and India but it is now made synthetically from napthalene. Henna and indigo together make Persian henna or henna reng which gives a strong blue-black colour.

Inorganic dyes

Inorganic dyes are based on the application of *metallic salts* to the hair. They include sulphide dyes, reduction dyes and the type formerly known as hair colour restorers. The presence of metallic salts such as those of lead, copper and silver on the hair can lead to difficulties if it is desired to perm the coloured hair later. The salts have molecules small enough to enter the hair shaft and often stay in the hair for a considerable time. Lead, copper and iron salts act as catalysts in the breakdown of hydrogen peroxide contained in perm neutralisers, and can produce enough heat to damage the hair. If it is suspected that hair has been treated with metallic dyes, it should be tested by immersing a strand from the hair in 6 per cent hydrogen peroxide. Bubbles of oxygen and heat indicate a metallic dye and processing involving the use of hydrogen peroxide should not be carried out on the hair.

Sulphide dyes or 'two-application' dyes
The hair is first treated with a solution of sodium sulphide, and then with

a solution of a metallic salt such as lead acetate, copper sulphate or silver nitrate. The corresponding metal sulphide is deposited both in the cortex and on the surface of the hair, e.g.

$$\begin{array}{cccc}
\text{sodium} & \text{copper} & \text{sodium} & \text{copper} \\
\text{sulphide} & + \text{sulphate} & = \text{sulphate} & + \text{sulphide} \\
& & \text{(washed away)} & \text{(deposited in} \\
& & & \text{the hair)}
\end{array}$$

Sodium sulphide should not be left on the hair alone as it acts as a depilatory.

Reduction dyes

Metallic salts, for example copper sulphate, may be reduced to the corresponding metal by the application of a reducing agent such as pyrogallol (trihydroxybenzene).

Experiment 9.2   Reduction dyes

Brush a 2 per cent solution of copper sulphate or cadmium sulphate on to a weft of blonde hair. Next dip the treated hair into a freshly prepared solution of alkaline 2 per cent pyrogallol. Rinse the hair and note the permanence of the dye.

'Hair colour restorers'

'Hair colour restorers' originally took the form of raw egg applied to the hair and combed through with a lead comb to form a deposit of lead sulphide.

Modern 'hair colour restorers' are used in home hairdressing but are not used professionally. They may be liquids or pomades containing lead acetate and sodium thiosulphate, which are applied daily to the hair until the desired shade is produced. The reaction between the two substances is very slow but black lead sulphide is gradually formed in the hair.

Experiment 9.3   'Hair colour restorers'

Make up the following solution:

Lead acetate	0.7 g
Sodium thiosulphate	1.8 g
Glycerol	5 ml
Water	95 ml

Prepare ten small bundles of blonde or light brown hair (or previously bleached hair) about 10 cm in length. Leave one bundle untreated as a control.

Day 1. Treat the other nine bundles with solution by using a brush or by dipping each bundle into the solution.

Day 2. Treat eight bundles only with solution.

Day 3. Treat only seven of the eight bundles with solution.

Continue in this manner each day until on day nine only one bundle remains to be treated. Compare the result for each day and note the build-up of colour. (WARNING – lead salts are poisonous.)

Synthetic organic dyes

These dyes, based on coal tar products such as aniline, form the most widely used group of dyes. They may be divided into the following three groups.

1. Temporary dyes

The molecules of temporary dyes are too large to enter the hair shaft unless the hair is very porous, so that they normally coat the outside of the hair shaft only. There are two types:

(a) **Cationic dyes** (basic dyes) such as methyl violet or methylene blue, which carry a positive charge and are therefore substantive to hair. They are water-soluble dyes obtainable in concentrated form to be diluted with water before application.

(b) **Anionic dyes** (acidic dyes) or azo dyes such as parahydroxyazobenzene.

The dyes may be applied as water rinses, colour shampoos, coloured plastic setting lotions or coloured lacquers, but all wash out at the first shampoo.

Water rinses are applied after shampooing and are dried on the hair. They are not successful in covering grey hair but are useful as complementary colours for removing unwanted 'off' colours, to brighten faded hair and to add highlights to grey hair. Cationic dyes are most useful on grey, white or bleached hair, usually adding slight blue or pink tones. Azo dyes give a good range of brown shades. Azo dyes are formulated with 90–95 per cent of citric or tartaric acid to give a pH of about 4. The hair may be rinsed with a 1 per cent solution of cetrimide, before application of the azo dye to reduce the negative charge on the hair which would tend to repel the dye. A setting lotion should not be used after a water rinse as it tends to remove some of the colour, leaving it patchy.

Colour shampoos contain azo dyes added to a soapless detergent, usually triethanolamine lauryl sulphate, along with a weak organic acid to give a pH of about 5 (see also Chapter 8).

Coloured plastic setting lotion is the most popular form of temporary colour. Azo dyes will combine chemically with plastic resins such as polyvinyl pyrrolidone, the dye molecules being attached at regular intervals along the long chain molecules of the resin. The coloured plastic is dissolved in isopropanol and water and applied as a setting lotion after shampooing. During hair drying the solvent evaporates, to leave a coloured plastic film on the hair.

Coloured lacquer also contains azo dyes combined with plastic resin dissolved in alcohol. The lacquer is sprayed, usually from an aerosol can, on to the dried hair after dressing out. A film of coloured resin is left on the hair when the solvent evaporates. Finely powdered aluminium is sometimes added to the spray to give lustre to the hair.

2. Semi-permanent colours

Semi-permanent colours consist of mixtures of *nitro dyes* which give red

and yellow colours, and *anthraquinones* which give blue colours, e.g.
(a) dinitro-amino-phenol (picramic acid) (red);
(b) nitro-phenylenediamine (yellow);
(c) tetra-amino-anthraquinone (blue).
The dyes are already in a coloured form and the molecules are small enough to enter the hair shaft. Mixtures of dyes of these three colours will produce a wide range of different shades, but the browns tend to be reddish or golden. Difficulties experienced with semi-permanent dyes are mostly due to the molecules of the red and yellow dyes being much smaller than those of the blue dyes. Thus if a brown dye is to be formulated from a mixture of all three colours, an excess of blue colour is usually added to ensure that sufficient of the larger blue molecules enter the hair shaft. If the hair is abnormally porous, for example, immediately after perming, more blue than usual will be absorbed and the colour balance upset. For this reason it is unwise to use a semi-permanent colour immediately after perming. Similarly the colours wash out and fade at different rates so that the colour on the hair changes with time.

Some of the dye molecules combine with the hydrogen bonds in keratin, and since the dye is not very soluble in water the colour gradually washes out in 6–8 shampoos, the dye in the hydrogen bonds being eventually replaced by water. The dyes are more soluble in detergent solution than in water so they are sometimes formulated with a shampoo base and used as a colour shampoo.

They are more often designed to be applied to dry hair as liquids or creams. Since they are not very soluble in water, a 'carrier' such as benzyl alcohol is added. This is a good solvent for the dye and acts as a dispersing agent which separates or disperses clusters of dye molecules, so aiding their penetration into the hair shafts. Cationic detergents are often added to ensure an even distribution of colour. Liquid preparations may be thickened by methyl cellulose. The speed of penetration of the dye into the hair can be increased by use of a steamer or infra-red heater.

3. Permanent oxidation dyes

Oxidation dyes are also known as *para dyes* since the earliest members of the group were para-phenylenediamine (black) and para-toluenediamine (brown). A wide range of other substances have since been added to the series. These include:-
(a) ortho-phenylenediamine (brown)
(b) para-aminophenol (reddish brown)
(c) ortho-aminophenol (light brown)
These oxidation bases are colourless or lightly coloured compounds which are soluble in water and have molecules small enough to enter the hair shaft. They are formulated as thick liquids or creams to be mixed with hydrogen peroxide (usually 6 per cent) immediately before use, the mixture being applied to the hair with a brush. The final colour of the dye is only reached by oxidation which takes place inside the hair cortex. Several small molecules combine to form larger molecules which are

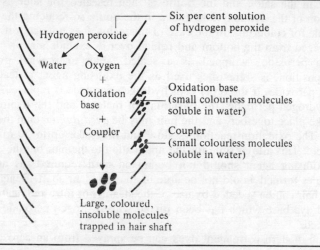

Fig 9.2 Permanent colour

insoluble in water. These larger molecules are coloured due to the re-arrangement of the atoms to form chromophores. The large, coloured, insoluble molecules form a permanent colour inside the hair shaft, though the colouring of the re-growth is necessary at intervals of 4–6 weeks if the colour is to be maintained.

In some cases, substances known as couplers are added to the oxidation bases to either modify or intensify the colour. Ash and blonde shades are usually produced by this method. During oxidation in the cortex, the couplers combine chemically with the oxidation bases to form much larger coloured molecules which are insoluble in water. These large coloured, insoluble molecules are trapped in the hair and do not wash out so that the dye is permanent (see Fig. 9.2). Meta-phenylenediamine is a coupler used with para-phenylenediamine to give grey-blue colours. Polyhydric phenols such as resorcinol and catechol are used as couplers with various oxidation bases to produce light brown and blonde shades.

The following substances are also added to the dye bases during manufacture:-

(a) Ammonium hydroxide, an alkali, added to give a pH of about 9. This makes the hair swell and allows easy entry of the dye into the hair. It also acts as a catalyst in the decomposition of hydrogen peroxide to produce oxygen for the oxidation process inside the hair.

(b) Lanolin, cetyl alcohol or glycerol is added as a conditioner.

(c) Triethanolamine oleate soap acts as a wetting agent and facilitates the rinsing of excess dye from the scalp.

(d) Sodium sulphite, a reducing agent, prevents premature oxidation of the dye bases in the tube or bottle during storage.

In order to avoid premature oxidation, the dye base is packed into sealed containers in an atmosphere of nitrogen. If only part of a bottle of dye is used in the salon and the bottle is then resealed for later use, some oxidation of the dye may take place in the bottle so reducing the amount available for colouring. In the case of tubes this does not occur if the tube is squeezed from the bottom and folded over to exclude air.

Urea peroxide, wrapped as a sealed tablet to prevent premature decomposition, is sometimes used as the oxidising agent instead of hydrogen peroxide. If the 6 per cent hydrogen peroxide is replaced by 9 per cent hydrogen peroxide, the bleaching of melanin and the dyeing of the hair take place together, and the hair may be *dyed lighter* than the natural shade. The oxidation reaction is slow and may take up to 30 minutes to complete. This allows time for the application to the hair but the dye base and oxidising agent should not be mixed until required, as any large molecules formed would not be able to enter the hair shaft. Reaction time on the hair can be speeded by use of the steamer or infra-red heaters. Any unused dye base which has been mixed with hydrogen peroxide must be discarded.

Some modern permanent dyes can be sprayed from an aerosol which contains two separate compartments, one containing the dye base and the other the hydrogen peroxide. The amount being dispensed from each compartment is controlled by a valve.

When the excess colour has been washed from the hair, a rinse containing *antioxidants* (reducing agents) and *acid* is beneficial. This stops further action by the hydrogen peroxide, neutralises excess alkali and closes the cuticle scales. Ascorbic acid, which is both a reducing agent and an acid, is often used for this purpose.

Para dyes have a good range of natural looking colours as well as fashion shades, and are easy to apply to the hair. Perming dyed hair leads to some loss of colour, and fading may occur if the hair is repeatedly subjected to strong sunlight.

Dangers in the use of para dyes

1. The most serious drawback to the use of para dyes is the danger of sensitisation to the dye, resulting in *dye dermatitis*. An allergic reaction to a dye may suddenly develop in a client who has been using the same dye over a long period of time. *A skin test* (also called patch test or hypersensitivity test) must be carried out 24 hours before each application of the dye. A positive reaction is indicated by redness, itching or blisters. Further contact with the dye must then be avoided and the area should be treated with calamine lotion or saline solution. Scalp injury caused by disease, physical or chemical damage may predispose a person to dye allergy (see also allergies in Chapter 3).

   The mildest symptoms of dye dermatitis are slight itching and erythema round the hair line. More severe symptoms may include swelling of the whole face including the lips. Men are often susceptible to para-dye dermatitis if the dye is used on the beard, since the skin of the face is more sensitive than that of the scalp. For this reason also, para dyes should not be used on the eyelashes or eyebrows.

2. Para dyes (and some semi permanent dyes) have been suspected of causing cancer.
3. Oxidation of the disulphide linkages could take place, causing chemical damage to the hair if a high percentage strength of hydrogen peroxide is used.

Quasi-permanent dyes

Mixtures of semi-permanent and oxidation dyes are often referred to as quasi-permanent dyes and are mixed with 3 or 6 per cent hydrogen peroxide immediately before application to the hair. The semi-permanent dye washes out gradually so the colour changes with time. As the permanent part of the dye remains, there is a problem of regrowth. A skin test is necessary before the use of these dyes.

The removal of unwanted colour

An undesirable but slight colour cast appearing in the hair as a result of colouring may be counteracted by the application of a dye which will absorb the light of the offending colour. For example, the green cast sometimes resulting from the application of a blue rinse to bleached hair may be counteracted by adding a small quantity of red pigment (usually as a water rinse). The red pigment absorbs the green light which would otherwise be reflected from the bleached hair.

The colour triangle of spectrum colours shows in Fig. 9.3 is useful in correcting colour casts. The offending colour is corrected by the addition of a small quantity of the colour opposite to it in the triangle.

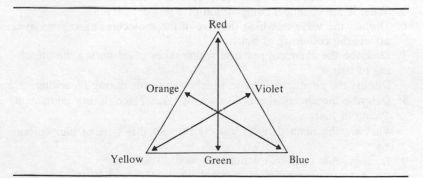

Fig 9.3 The colour triangle

The total removal of unwanted dyes on the hair is a more difficult process, and to avoid hair damage a strand test should be carried out first on a sample cut from the hair.

Oxidation dyes may be removed by applying one of the following to the hair.

1. A solution of 20 parts of 6 per cent hydrogen peroxide mixed with 1 part of 0.88 ammonium hydroxide.
2. A 5 per cent solution of sodium hydrosulphite (a reducing agent).
3. A 6 per cent solution of sodium formaldehyde sulphoxalate (a reducing agent).
   Semi-permanent dyes may be removed by
(a) washing vigorously with shampoo to which a few drops of 0.88 ammonium hydroxide have been added;
(b) spirit soap (4 parts soft soap to 1 part alcohol).

Metallic dyes are best left to grow out with the hair but some metallic dyes are removed by an acidified 2 per cent solution of sodium thiosulphate. A strand test is required.

Questions

1. Why is henna known as a progressive dye?
   Describe the effect of the addition to henna of;
   (a) acetic acid;   (b) a mild alkali.
2. Why may an unwanted green cast appear on the bleached hair after use of a toner?
   What procedure would you adopt to correct the colour?
3. Explain the meaning of: (a) nascent oxygen;
   (b) a catalyst;   (c) an oxidising agent.
4. What is meant by a bleach booster?
   Give one example of a substance used as a booster.
5. What is the chemical composition of a powder bleach?
6. Discuss the ways in which the size of the molecules of various dyes affects the colouring of hair.
7. Describe the chemical reaction which takes place during the bleaching of hair.
   Discuss the chemical damage which may occur during bleaching.
8. Describe the chemical reaction which takes place during permanent dyeing of hair.
   What are the main dangers associated with this type of hair colouring?
9. Discuss what course of action you would take:
   (a) if you suspected that a client desiring a cold perm, had been previously treating her hair with metallic dyes;
   (b) to ensure that hair remained in good condition after a permanent tint;
   (c) if a client asked to have a semi-permanent colour removed from her hair;
   (d) if a patch test, taken before application of a permanent dye, proved positive.

10. (a) What are the qualities of a good dye?
    (b) Explain the meaning of: (i) quasi permanent dyes; (ii) bleach toners.

    List the chemicals which may be found in each, and discuss any precautions which should be taken in their use.

Chapter 10

Waving and straightening hair

Reasons for curl

The reasons for natural waviness or straightness of hair are not fully
understood, though various theories have been suggested.

1. The amount of curl depends on the cross-section of the hair. Wavy hair
   was considered to be oval, straight hair round and kinky, negroid type
   hair kidney shaped in cross-section. This theory has now been dis-
   counted.
2. Curl depends on the shape of the follicle. A straight follicle produces
   straight hair and a curved follicle a curly hair.
3. Curl is caused by a difference in structure between one side of a
   hair compared with the other, giving rise to a 'para' and an 'ortho'
   cortex (see Fig. 10.1).

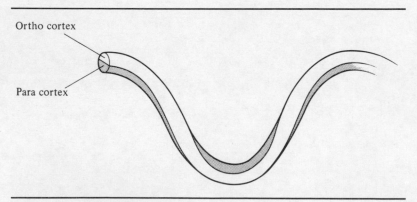

Fig 10.1 The ortho and para cortex

This dual cortex can be detected in very curly hair by certain staining
techniques followed by microscopic examination of cross-sections of
hairs. The ortho cortex has a less dense structure and a lower sulphur
content than the para cortex and always lies on the outside of the wave.
The structure may be compared to that of a straight hair which has been
permanently waved. The hair on the outer curve is stretched (therefore
less dense) and that of the inner surface is compressed.

Setting

The straightening of wavy or curly hair, and the waving or curling of straight hair, involve the same processes. The required changes may be brought about in two ways:

1. **By physical changes** involving the mechanical shaping of the hair, producing a temporary set.
2. **By chemical changes** to the structure of keratin, producing a permanent set.

Temporary setting

Temporary setting can be carried out as a *cohesive set* or as a *heat set*. The sets are easily destroyed by cold water in the case of a cohesive set and hot water in the case of a heat set.

Cohesive set

During a normal 'shampoo and set' using methods such as roller setting, blow drying, water waving and pin curling, a cohesive set is produced. To obtain a good long-lasting set the following requirements are necessary:

1. The hair must be in good condition and therefore be strongly elastic. Overprocessed hair, bleached hair or very dry hair lacks elasticity and will not produce a good set.
2. The hair must be wet to soften it and to obtain maximum extension during setting. The hair is usually shampooed before setting, the detergent acting as a wetting agent which brings the water into closer contact with the hair.
3. Tension must be applied to stretch the hair into the desired shape, e.g. by winding the hair tightly round the roller or by use of a brush in blow-drying or comb in water waving.
4. The hair must be thoroughly dried whilst the stretching force is maintained. (If rollers are removed before the hair is dry there will be some loss of set.) On completion of drying the hair remains 'set' in its new position even when the stretching force is removed.

The mechanism of setting

Hair is elastic due to the coiled spring arrangement of the polypeptide chains in the keratin of the cortical fibres. It will stretch if pulled and then spring back when released. In dry hair the amount of stretching is limited mainly by hydrogen bonds which hold together the coils of the chains (see Fig. 10.2) and also to some extent by the cross linkages between adjacent chains. Although the hydrogen bonds are individually weak, they are very numerous and so are effective in restricting the amount of stretching. The scales of the cuticle will slip over each other during

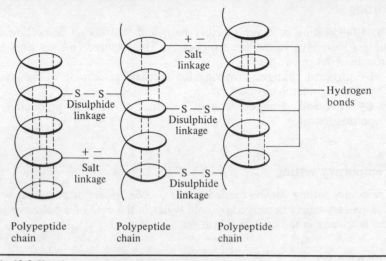

Fig 10.2 Keratin structure showing numerous hydrogen bonds

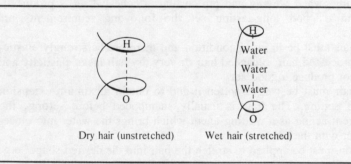

Dry hair (unstretched)   Wet hair (stretched)

Fig 10.3 Bound water in a hydrogen bond

stretching so they do not prevent the extension of the hair.

When hair is wet, some of the water molecules join the hydrogen bonds to form '*bound water*' (see Fig. 10.3). This allows a greater extension of the hair to take place in wet hair than in dry hair, therefore wet hair produces the better set.

The keratin of unstretched hair is known as *alpha-keratin* (α keratin). When wet hair is stretched, the polypeptide chains straighten out to form *beta-keratin* (β keratin). If hair is dried whilst still being stretched, the bound water evaporates and the hydrogen and oxygen atoms of the original hydrogen bonds are left too far apart to re-form the bonds (see Fig. 10.4). New hydrogen bonds are formed and these hold the fibre in the stretched position. Therefore, when the stretching force e.g. the roller, is removed, the hair remains set in its stretched state.

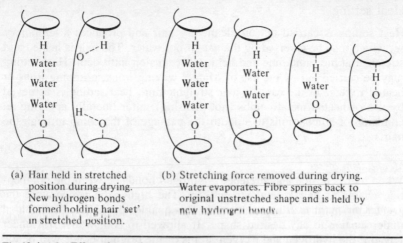

(a) Hair held in stretched
position during drying.
New hydrogen bonds
formed holding hair 'set'
in stretched position.

(b) Stretching force removed during drying.
Water evaporates. Fibre springs back to
original unstretched shape and is held by
new hydrogen bonds.

Fig 10.4(a)(b) Effect of removing stretching force during drying

If, however, the stretching force is removed before the hair is dry and
drying is completed without tension, the bound water evaporates and the
fibre springs back to its natural spiral shape. New hydrogen bonds are
formed to hold it in the unstretched shape (see Fig. 10.4*a, b*).

Loss of set
If 'set' hair is wetted again and then allowed to dry without tension, the
set is lost and the hair reverts to the unstretched α-keratin state. Hair is
hygroscopic and in Britain the absorption of moisture from humid air is
usually sufficient to cause gradual loss of set, whereas in very dry areas of
the world a set may last for a considerable time. Excessive scalp perspiration may also cause loss of set. The absorption of moisture is reduced
by the natural coating of sebum on the hair, and this may be assisted
artificially by the application of setting lotions, dressing creams and
lacquer.

The level of humidity of the air in salons themselves should be carefully controlled by good ventilation. A wall hygrometer is useful to
indicate relative humidity, which should not exceed 70 per cent.

Danger of damage to hair during cohesive setting
1. Use of spiked rollers during setting may cause splitting of the hair
   shaft.
2. The frequent use of brush rollers or excessively tight rollers may cause
   traction alopecia especially at the front margin.
3. The hair cuticle may be damaged if the hot nozzle of a blow dryer is
   allowed to touch the hair.
4. The abrasive effect of brushing wet hair as in blow drying quickly
   erodes the cuticle scales and is more damaging than brushing dry hair.

Heat setting

Heat setting is carried out on clean, dry hair and produces a temporary set which may be reversed by the use of hot water. The hair is heated and stretched at the same time and held under tension until cool. Heat setting may be carried out by the use of Marcel waving irons, crimping irons or heated rollers. In the case of hair straightening, heat setting is achieved by use of heated metal combs (hot pressing), after liberally applying an emulsion of silicone oils to smooth the passage of the comb through the hair.

Mechanism of set

When hair is heated and stretched, hydrogen bonds between the polypeptide chains of hair keratin are broken. The higher the temperature the greater the number of broken bonds. This enables the hair to be moulded under tension to any desired shape. If allowed to cool whilst still under tension, the hydrogen and oxygen atoms of the original bonds will be too far apart to re-form the old bonds, but will form new bonds with other atoms close by. The new bonds keep the hair in its new set shape.

Destruction of the set

The set is destroyed if the hair is wetted with water of approximately the same temperature as that used in setting. The new hydrogen bonds will be broken, and if the hair then dries without tension, the original bonds will be restored. Cold water will not remove the set as too few of the new hydrogen bonds would be broken at that temperature.

Danger of damage to hair by heat setting

1. Repeated heating damages the cuticle, making the hair rough and therefore lacking in lustre. It becomes subject to static electricial charges on brushing or combing, leading to fly-away hair.
2. If the irons are too hot the cuticle may be damaged or the whole hair burnt, resulting in breakage.
3. Burns to the scalp can cause damage to the hair roots and subsequent bald patches.
4. Traction alopecia, especially at the front margins of the hair, may result from heat and repeated pulling by the comb during hair straightening. This is particularly liable to happen when dealing with negroid type hair, which is difficult to comb due to the tightness of the curl.

Permanent setting

Permanent setting involves chemical changes to the disulphide linkages of keratin. The changes take place during cold perming, tepid perming, heat perming and hair straightening. A permanent set cannot be removed by wetting with water at any temperature.

Pre-perm treatment

After examining the scalp for cuts or inflammation and following a pre-perm shampoo to remove grease, a protein filler or conditioner may be used before commencing the perm. Protein fillers contain protein hydrolysates (see Chapter 7) or mixtures of amino acids, dipeptides and short chains of amino acids. The hydrolysates are substantive to hair, becoming attached electrostatically to both free acid groups and free basic groups in the hair. The filler helps to prevent the loss of amino acids which takes place during perming, and therefore leaves the hair in good condition when perming is completed.

Cold permanent waving

Cold waving takes place in two distinct stages:

1. **The application of cold wave lotion** and winding of the hair on to curlers where the chemical process of reduction takes place. This causes some of the cystine linkages of keratin to break, whilst the hair is softened and takes the shape of the curler.
2. **The application of the neutraliser.** The chemical process of oxidation takes place involving the rebuilding of the cystine linkages into a new position on the polypeptide chain, thus holding the hair in the desired shape.

Reagents used in cold waving

Cold wave lotion. The main active ingredient of cold wave lotion is ammonium thioglycollate (also called ammonium thiolethanoate), a salt which is also a *reducing agent*. The salt is manufactured by the neutralisation of thioglycollic acid (mercapto-acetic acid or thiolethanoic acid) by ammonium hydroxide.

thioglycollic acid	+	ammonium hydroxide	=	ammonium thioglycollate	+	water
acid	+	alkali	=	a salt	+	water

Monoethanolamine thioglycollate is sometimes used instead of ammonium thioglycollate as it has a less objectionable smell.

The other ingredients of the lotion are:

(a) ammonium hydroxide which is added in excess of that required to neutralise the thioglycollic acid, to give a pH of 9.5;
(b) alkanolamides (non-ionic detergents) to act as wetting agents;
(c) protein hydrolysates or cetrimide as a conditioner;
(d) silicone fluids which increase the life of the perm;
(e) ammonium chloride or ammonium carbonate may be added as a buffer;
(f) colour and perfume.

The lotion may be formulated as a thin clear liquid, or as an emulsion cream which is easier to control on the hair. The cream is an oil-in-water emulsion containing about 10 per cent mineral oil, with cetyl alcohol as the emulsifying agent. The oil is used only as a thickening agent, and the emulsion must be particularly stable or oil would be deposited on the hair and prevent the entry of the active ingredients.

The neutraliser. The 'neutraliser' used in cold waving is in fact an *oxidising agent* such as hydrogen peroxide or sodium bromate, though sodium perborate is sometimes used for home perms. The neutraliser may be formulated as a liquid or a cream.

Liquid types contain either a 6 per cent solution of hydrogen peroxide or a 5 per cent solution of sodium bromate, with 1 per cent soapless detergent added to produce a foam which holds the neutraliser in place on the hair. *Cream types* are oil-in-water emulsions mixed with 6 per cent hydrogen peroxide solution immediately before use.

Chemical reactions taking place during cold waving

Small sections of hair are damped with the lotion and wound on to curlers *without tension*, or if winding is carried out quickly the whole head may be damped with lotion before winding (pre-saturation). Ammonium hydroxide (an alkali) in the lotion makes the hair swell, and acts as a wetting agent to allow easy penetration of the lotion into the cortex. The hydrogen bonds and salt linkages of the hair are broken in the alkaline solution. The reducing agent, ammonium thioglycollate, supplies hydrogen atoms which become attached to the sulphur atoms in the disulphide linkages lying between the polypeptide chain of hair keratin. This breaks the bond between the sulphur atoms and each molecule of cystine forms two molecules of the amino acid cysteine (see Fig. 10.5). This chemical reaction, which involves the addition of hydrogen to a substance, is known as reduction. Each molecule of cysteine contains a thiol or mercaptan group (– SH).

Reduction is speeded by heat, and a plastic cap covering the head retains sufficient body heat for the purpose. Whilst the keratin is in a reduced state with many linkages broken, the hair may be damaged if subjected to tension. The breakage of the linkages enables the hair to be moulded to the shape of the curlers, the polypeptide chains moving in

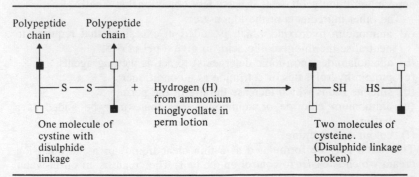

Fig 10.5 The process of reduction in cold waving

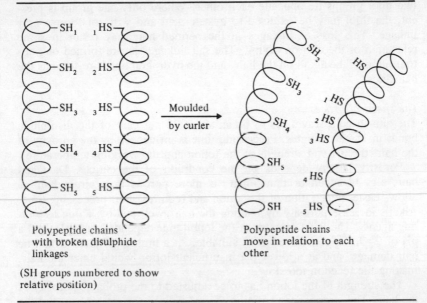

Fig 10.6 Moulding the hair to the shape of the curler

relation to each other (see Fig. 10.6). When a satisfactory curl has been obtained, the cold wave lotion is rinsed from the hair with the curlers still in position.

Neutralising is then carried out. This is an oxidation process and not chemical neutralisation. Oxygen is produced from the oxidising agent, either hydrogen peroxide or sodium borate, in the neutraliser. The oxygen removes hydrogen atoms from the cysteine molecules to form water, so allowing adjacent sulphur atoms to join together to rebuild disulphide linkages in a different position along the polypeptide chains. The new linkages hold the hair permanently in its new shape (see Fig. 10.7).

The re-forming of the disulphide linkages can only take place when

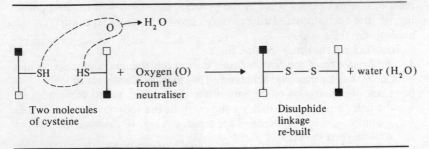

Fig 10.7 Oxidation to reform disulphide linkages in a new position on the polypeptide chains

two thiol groups lie opposite each other. Where only one group is present, the thiol may be oxidised to cysteic acid and will not form a new linkage. This loss of linkages in the permed hair may result in some relaxation of the curl on drying. The salt linkages are re-formed on neutralisation of the alkali on the hair, and the hydrogen bonds re-form as the hair dries.

The speed of processing

The aim in cold waving is to break about 20 per cent of the disulphide bonds in 15–20 minutes. Processing time is influenced by the porosity of the hair, the pH and strength of the lotion and the working temperature.

Porosity largely depends on the condition of the cuticle. Damaged hair, e.g. bleached or tinted hair, is more porous than virgin hair so allows easier penetration of the lotion and requires short processing time. Alkalis increase porosity by making the hair swell and by acting as wetting agents. The level of entry of the lotion thus depends on its pH, and a pH of 9–9.5 is considered most suitable. At a higher pH there would be hair damage, and at a lower pH insufficient lotion would enter the hair, making the reaction too slow.

The strength of the lotion has to be adjusted to the probable porosity of the hair. The stronger the solution the more linkages are broken, but the more resistant the hair the less solution enters the cortex. Thus 8–10 per cent ammonium thioglycollate solutions are used for virgin hair, 6–8 per cent solution for average hair and 5–6 per cent solutions for tinted or bleached hair. If on examination of a test curl during processing time the lotion appears to be working too slowly, the hair may be re-damped with a stronger solution. If it appears to be working too quickly the reaction may be slowed by damping with de-ionised water.

Most perm lotions are designed to work at a salon temperature of 20–22 °C when the hair is covered with a plastic cap to retain the heat of the scalp. Colder conditions may make the reaction too slow.

Reasons for failure in cold waving

Cold waving is a balance between the number of disulphide linkages broken by reduction, and the number re-formed during oxidation. If this balance is upset at any point of the process, the result will be disappointing if not disastrous. Failure may involve insufficient curl or an excessively tight curl.

Insufficient curl may be due to

1. *The breakage of too few linkages* during the reduction process so that a new shape cannot be achieved. This may be the result of
   (a) Lack of penetration of the lotion into the cortex, due to substances on the hair, e.g. grease blocking the entry of the lotion, use of a low pH lotion, e.g. a lotion intended for tepid waving, or resistant hair with a well-aligned cuticle.
   (b) Use of a lotion which is too weak for the type of hair, e.g. use on virgin hair of a lotion intended for average use.

(c) Insufficient processing time.

(d) Coldness of the surroundings.

2. *The breakage of too many disulphide linkages* by using a strong lotion on porous hair, an over-long processing time or an abnormally high salon temperature. If too many linkages are broken, neutralising may not be completely effective and the hair will not hold its new shape.

3. *Under-neutralising.* If neutralising is omitted or is insufficient, or if the curlers are removed before neutralising is completed, gradual oxidation of the linkages will take place in the air but they will no longer be re-formed in the desired position. In order to maintain the desired shape, the hair must be held in the required position until the new linkages are formed.

4. *Over-neutralising.* Excessive oxidation may change cysteine to cysteic acid which will not form cross linkages. Thus the number of disulphide linkages may be considerably reduced, resulting in lack of curl and weakening of the hair. Over-neutralising may be caused by leaving the neutraliser on the hair too long, or by the use of a solution of oxidising agent which is too strong.

Excessively tight curl may or may not be desired. Permed hair may have a very tight curl due to the use of

1. Small diameter curlers. The size of the curler determines the diameter of the curl (see Fig. 10.8). It is possible to change the curler size quickly during the reduction process if it is thought to be wrong. The curl is not made permanent until neutralising has been carried out.

2. A lotion which is too strong for the type of hair.

3. An over-long processing time.

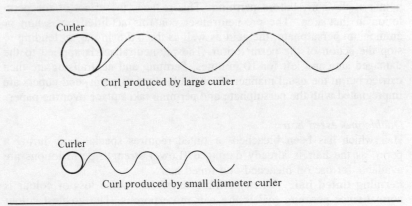

Fig 10.8 Tightness of curl

Modifications of cold waving

The search for methods of permanent waving which leave the hair in good condition, and a general move against the use of strongly alkaline materials has led to the introduction of many modifications to traditional cold waving.

Perm lotions which are slightly alkaline or even slightly acid have been developed and rely on heat to open the cuticle scales, along with wetting agents to ensure adequate penetration of the lotion into the cortex. The amount of heat required is not as great as that for true heat perms so this type is known as a tepid perm. Heat may be applied by a conventional hood dryer, by infra-red dryers or by heated plastic clips applied to each curl. The lotion may contain ammonium thioglycollate, monoethanolamine thioglycollate or ammonium sulphite as the reducing agent though glyceryl monothioglycollate is now often used for acid perms. When the desired curl has been achieved the hair is rinsed with water and neutralised as in cold waving. Large diameter curlers are often used to give a casual but not very long lasting curl. This type of perm is particularly useful for hair which is already in poor condition.

To improve the condition of limp hair a citric acid rinse is sometimes included between the reduction and oxidation processes. This neutralises any alkali left on the hair and increases its elasticity, leaving the hair in better condition for setting. Sodium bromate is used as the oxidising agent, as release of oxygen from hydrogen peroxide is inhibited by acid conditions.

So–called 'moisturising' perms intended for use on dry hair contain humecants or water-attracting substances designed to make the hair more elastic. Glycerine and polyvinyl pyrrolidone (PVP) are used in this way. Protein hydrolysates are also added to perm lotions and neutralisers as conditioners.

For the uniform perming of damaged hair a 'pre-neutralising' agent or acidified oxidising agent is applied to the damaged portion, usually the points of the hair, before perming. This reduces the effect of the perm lotion in that area. The pre-neutraliser contains acidified potassium or ammonium persulphate, the acid as well as the oxidising agent tending to stop the action of the perm lotion. The pre-neutraliser is applied to the damaged area and left for 10 minutes. Perming and neutralising are then carried out in the usual manner. In a similar type of perm, end papers are impregnated with the persulphate and perming takes place over the paper.

Double processed hair

Hair which has been bleached or tinted requires special care during a perm, as the hair is already damaged. Lower strength perm lotions are available for use on bleached and tinted hair.

Perming tinted hair. When perming tinted hair some loss of colour is normal since perming makes the hair more porous. The greatest colour loss takes place during the rinse before neutralising, and omission of this rinse will minimise the loss. The perm processing time should however be slightly reduced to allow for the continued action of the perm lotion left in the hair.

If it is desired to both perm and tint on the same occasion, tinting may be carried out first but allowance must be made for the loss of colour during perming, and the pre-neutralising rinse should be omitted. Alternatively perming may be carried out before tinting, adjusting the tint for the probable increased intensity of the colour on newly permed hair. Tints can be manufactured as part of neutralising solutions so that neutralising and tinting may procede together, but these are little used.

Perming bleached hair. A high proportion (up to about 50 per cent) of disulphide linkages may be destroyed during bleaching. This means that when wetted with perm lotion bleached hair quickly absorbs a large quantity of the lotion, which is drawn up in the spaces between the polypeptide chains, forcing them apart. The effect may be partly overcome by wetting the hair with water only before winding, and applying the lotion when winding is completed. Thus the progress of the perm may be carefully watched as the processing time will be short.

Further loss of disulphide linkages will take place during perming and hair breakage could occur. For bleached hair in very poor condition, a strand test should be carried out to check the effect of perming before proceeding. Perm lotions based on monoethanolamine are useful on bleached hair as they have a lower pH than lotions based on ammonium hydroxide. Perming may not be successful on bleached hair if too many disulphide linkages were already lost during bleaching.

Dangers associated with cold perming

The damage caused by cold perming may affect the hair, skin or eyes.

Damage to the hair. The number of disulphide linkages in hair is always reduced by perming. This loss is increased by incorrect procedures; that is, by excessive bond breakage during reduction or over-oxidation whilst neutralising. Some oxidation products are soluble so loss of protein always takes place during perming, especially from the matrix of twisted polypeptide chains between the cortical fibres. Fragments of the cuticle may also break off whilst the hair is swollen. Decrease in the number of linkages causes loss of tensile strength and elasticity. The hair thus becomes weaker, more porous, and has a greater tendency to split after being permed.

Tension applied to the hair during perming but before neutralising may lead to hair breakage. Such damage may occur if the hair has been wound too tightly, if the hair is pulled, or if the curler elastic presses on the hair or is twisted over the hair. Hair breakage may also occur if the hair has already been weakened by previous treatment such as bleaching, or if the pH of the lotion is greater than 9.5. If the lotion is allowed on to the scalp and enters the follicles between the outer root sheath and the hair, the extra warmth of the head may increase the speed of reaction and cause hair breakage.

During neutralising, breakage may occur if the hair has been previously treated with iron or copper salts. These act as catalysts in the breakdown of the hydrogen peroxide in the neutraliser and sufficient heat may be given out to cause hair breakage (see metallic dyes in Chapter 9). In contact with iron salts, perm lotion itself produces a purple coloured compound which may discolour fair hair.

Damage to the skin. Perm lotion can cause chemical burns and contact dermatitis so should be applied to the hair only. It should not be allowed to run on to the skin or into the client's ears which are particularly susceptible to dermatitis. Cotton wool should not be placed round the hairline during the application of perm lotion as this quickly becomes saturated and holds the lotion in contact with the skin. The hairdresser should wear rubber gloves during perming.

Damage to the eyes. If perm lotion enters the eye, severe irritation may be caused. The eye should be rinsed immediately using a large quantity of warm water poured gently over the eye from a jug. Care should be taken not to wash the lotion into the undamaged eye.

After perm treatment

1. An acid rinse after perming is completed will neutralise any alkali remaining on the hair and reduce the swelling of the hair caused by the alkali. Acids also tend to stop the action of the oxidising agent in the neutraliser. Ascorbic acid is often used after perming as it is both an acid and a reducing agent, and so is effective in stopping the action of hydrogen peroxide. Acids also precipitate any soluble oxidation products which may have formed in the cortex during perming, and so prevent loss of protein material from the hair.

2. Conditioners of the cetrimide type which are substantive to hair are useful after perming, as they are taken up to a greater extent if the hair is damaged and remain effective even after rinsing.

3. The curl produced by perming is often too tight for many styles, and the hair is usually cohesively set on rollers of larger diameter.

Heat perming

Typical ingredients of a heat perm lotion are as follows:

0.88 ammonium hydroxide	20%	(an alkali)
Borax	5%	(an alkaline salt)
Sodium or potassium sulphite	2%	(a reducing agent)
Water	73%	

The hair is first shampooed to remove grease and lacquer which would reduce the penetration of the lotion into the cortex. The lotion is applied to the hair which is *wound fairly tightly* on to curlers. Some form of heat must then be applied. Early methods of heating included *electrical heaters* which were attached to each curl (spiral winding), and *steam processing*. In *falling-heat* or wire-less methods, metal clips heated by conduction on electrically heated bars are placed over the curls. To prevent burns, the scalp is insulated by slipping a rubber pad under each curl. In the modern equivalent of this method the clips are plastic instead of metal, but are heated in a similar manner though to a lower temperature (see tepid waving). Another method of heating is by *exothermic pads* containing calcium oxide (quicklime). Each pad is dipped into cold water before being applied – one pad to each curl. The chemical reaction between calcium oxide and water produces heat and is therefore said to be an *exothermic reaction*.

calcium oxide   +   water ⟶ calcium hydroxide +   heat
(a basic oxide)   (an alkali)

The chemical pads or sachets become hot enough to burn the skin so must not touch the client's scalp. Chemical burns could result if the calcium oxide powder from the pad is allowed to come into contact with the skin. The pads should be kept in an air-tight tin since they absorb moisture from the air, gradually forming calcium hydroxide.

Chemical reactions taking place during heat perming
In heat perms some disulphide linkages are broken by sodium or potassium sulphite, which are only effective as reducing agents at about 60 °C. Most of the linkages however are broken by the chemical process of *hydrolysis* due to the action of the alkali, ammonium hydroxide. Hydrolysis means the decomposition of a substance with the elements of water being added to the substances formed during the decomposition. Thus in heat perming cystine is decomposed and the elements of water are added to the substances formed (see Fig. 10.9).

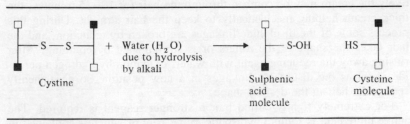

Fig 10.9 Cystine linkage broken by hydrolysis

More complex reactions are also known to take place during the breakdown of disulphide linkages in heat perming. The breakage of the disulphide linkages allows the realignment of the peptide chains and the hair takes the shape of the curler. The chemical action continues with the reforming of some linkages, one type of new cross linkage being a sulphide linkage (containing only one sulphur atom) which is part of the amino acid lanthionine (see Fig. 10.10). Water and hydrogen sulphide

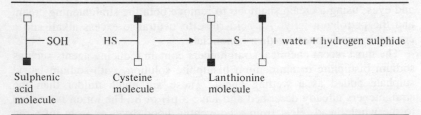

Fig 10.10 Continuation of chemical action with formation of lanthionine

gas (which smells of bad egg) are produced during this latter part of the reaction.

The hair may be tightly wound on the curlers as the hair is never in such a delicate state as in cold waving. In heat perming the chemical reaction is continuous and there is no separation between bond breaking and bond re-forming.

The heated clips or pads are left in place on the hair until they cool. After removal, the lotion is rinsed from the hair, which is then ready to take a cohesive set.

Permanent straightening of hair

Permanent setting or chemical straightening of hair can be carried out using the same reagents and processes as in the curling of straight hair by cold perming. The straightening agent is a much thicker oil-in-water emulsion than that used in cold wave lotions and the concentration of ammonium thioglycollate is higher. Straightening creams contain 10–12 per cent of ammonium thioglycollate and have a pH of 10. After application of the cream, the hair is wound on to large diameter rollers. Alternatively the cream may be combed through the hair for 10–15 minutes, the thick cream helping mechanically to keep the hair straight. During this process some of the disulphide linkages are broken by reduction, and the hair takes the shape of the rollers or is straightened by combing. After rinsing away the reducing agent with water, oxidation by hydrogen peroxide re-forms the disulphide linkages in a new position, so permanently setting the hair in the desired shape.

For extremely tightly curled hair a stronger reagent is required. The active ingredient is sodium hydroxide, 5 per cent of which is contained in an oil-in-water emulsion with about 40 per cent of fatty material. The thick cream is combed through the hair for a short time, the strong alkali breaking the disulphide linkages by hydrolysis. The manufacturers' instructions must be carefully followed, as overprocessing can lead to complete destruction of the hair. The cream is caustic and must not be allowed to touch either the client's scalp or the hairdresser's hands. The skin of the scalp must be protected by application of petroleum jelly before using the cream. After straightening is completed, the cream must be rinsed off at a back wash basin to avoid damage to the client's skin and eyes, using a cream shampoo to remove both the straightening cream and the petroleum jelly. An acid rinse to neutralise excess alkali and a cetrimide conditioner are then beneficial.

The most recent chemical straighteners contain reducing agents such as sodium bisulphite or ammonium bisulphite solution, with sodium lauryl sulphate added as a wetting agent. These are much milder than the straighteners already described and have a pH of 8. The lotion is applied to the whole head. Heat from a convential hood dryer or from infra-red lamps is applied for 15 minutes to speed the chemical reaction during which cystine linkages are reduced to cysteine. The hair is then combed straight for 15 minutes. After rinsing off the lotion oxidation is carried out, using hydrogen peroxide solution to re-form the cystine linkages which sets the hair in the new straight position.

Dangers of chemical straightening

Thioglycollate straighteners are more likely to cause scalp irritation than the lotions used for cold waving, since they are more concentrated and have a higher pH value. If combing methods are used there is also more contact with the scalp. They should not be used on clients with sensitive skins, or if there are cuts and abrasions, or if any inflamation is present on the scalp.

They are also more damaging to the hair. Breakage may take place during combing when the hair is in its weakened reduced state before neutralising has been carried out. A wide-toothed comb should be used to avoid excessive tension on the hair. Straighteners should not be used on hair which is in poor condition, or has been previously tinted or bleached or is already damaged by frequent hot pressing.

Sodium hydroxide-based creams are caustic and have a depilatory action if contact time with the hair is too great. The danger of breakage by combing is greater than during the use of thioglycollate straighteners.

Products used to preserve a cohesive set

A cohesive set is destroyed if moisture enters the hair shaft. Substances such as setting lotions, lacquers and dressing creams which coat the hair with a moisture-resisting film thus help to preserve the set.

Setting lotions

Setting lotions are sprayed on to the wet hair after shampooing and before setting. They keep the hair damp during setting, so increasing elasticity and facilitating the stretching of the hair. They also make the set last longer by coating the hair with a protective film when dry. The lotions are solutions containing *a film-former* dissolved in a suitable *solvent* which evaporates and leaves the film-former on the hair.

The film-formers are either *natural gums* or *synthetic resins*. Gums are carbohydrates which when mixed with water form a sticky solution or mucilage. Gums are obtained from certain trees by damaging the bark. The gum forms an exudation from the wound and is picked off the tree by hand. Since it is a natural product, the composition and purity varies. Gum tragacanth is a white powder obtained from Turkey. Gum Karaya, from India, is cheaper and gives a softer film than gum tragacanth. Gum arabic, from Senegal, may also be used.

Gums have largely been replaced in modern setting lotions by synthetic resins. These are polymers consisting of long chain molecules made by linking together many smaller molecules of the same type (or in the case of co-polymers, two or more different types of molecule), during a chemical reaction known as polymerisation.

The following resins are commonly used as film formers.

1. *Polyvinyl pyrrolidone* (PVP) is soluble in both water and alcohol, and is easily shampooed from the hair. It is substantive to hair, is antistatic and gives the hair a soft feel by attracting moisture. This hygroscopic quality has the disadvantage that the film becomes soft and sticky in humid conditions. In a dry atmosphere it tends to be brittle and flaky. These disadvantages are overcome by forming a co-polymer with polyvinyl acetate (PVA or Gelva resin). PVA is insoluble in water but soluble in alcohol. It is not substantive to hair nor is it hygroscopic. The copolymer prepared in the proportion of 60 per cent PVP and 40 per cent PVA gives a firmer hold than PVP alone, is soluble in water and substantive to hair like PVP but is resistant to humidity.

2. *Dimethyl hydantoin formaldehyde* (DMHF) is soluble in both water and alcohol and is easily shampooed from the hair. The film is glossy but brittle, and the addition of a plasticiser is essential to soften the film. DMHF is slightly hygroscopic and the hair can be reset using a wet comb or brush.

The solvents for setting lotions are usually mixtures of water and some form of alcohol such as ethanol, industrial methylated spirit or isopropanol.

The main additives to setting lotions are

(a) plasticisers, usually glycerol, added to keep the dry film soft and pliable;

(b) preservative such as formaldehyde which is necessary in gum setting lotions to prevent the growth of moulds;

(c) conditioners such as protein hydrolysates;

(d) colour;

(e) perfume.

The formulation of setting lotions

Gum setting lotions contain 1 per cent of gum dissolved in industrial methylated spirit and water with small quantities of glycerol as a plasticiser, and formaldehyde as a preservative. Some gum setting lotions contain alkalis such as borax or triethanolamine, to soften the hair and so make it easier to set.

Plastic setting lotions contain 1–2 per cent resin dissolved in industrial spirit and water, with glycerol as a plasticiser. Heat styling setting lotions designed for use during blow drying, and hair straightening by hot combs, often contain (in addition to plastic resins) protein hydrolysates and silicone oils to give the hair a smoother surface and so lessen friction between the hair and the brush or comb. Silicone oils produce a heat-resistant film which helps to prevent damage by the blow dryer.

Coloured setting lotions (see also Chapter 9) contain azo dyes joined chemically into the polymer chains of PVP/VA resins. The setting lotions are formulated in the same way as uncoloured setting lotions.

Aerosol foam setting lotions produce foam as the product is leaving the aerosol can, but the foam is designed to be unstable and soon breaks down on the hair. The setting lotion is based on plastic resins in a detergent solution. The aerosol propellant which forces the ingredients from the can is usually a fluorinated hydrocarbon. This vaporises as it leaves the can, the vapour creating bubbles as it passes through the detergent solution.

Lacquers

Lacquers are applied to the dry hair by the use of aerosol sprays or puffer sprays, after the dressing is completed. They are designed to keep the hair in position and to protect the set by preventing the absorption of moisture (see Fig. 10.11). Like setting lotions, lacquers consist of a film-former dissolved in a suitable solvent but they contain less water as they are used on dry, set hair.

A good lacquer should dry quickly, leaving a tough, clear, flexible, colourless, adhesive film which should not become tacky in a humid

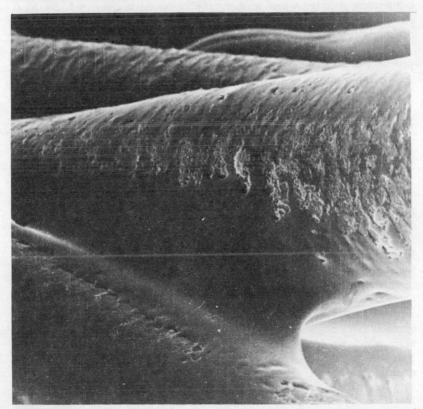

Fig 10.11 How hairspray holds hairs together, thereby maintaining the style

atmosphere or flake in a dry atmosphere. It should be easy to wash from the hair and be non-toxic and non-irritant to the skin. Lacquers should be kept out of client's eyes and off the skin as they can cause dermatitis. Although lacquers have not been proved to be responsible for any particular damage to the lungs or the lining of the nose and throat, it is wise to avoid inhaling them on grounds of general health.

The film-formers used in lacquers are either shellac, a natural resin, or synthetic plastic resins. The holding power of the lacquer, that is the firmness or softness of hold, depends on the nature of the film-former, its concentration and degree of plasticity.

Shellac is produced by the female lac insect (Laccifer lacca) to surround her eggs which are laid on the bark of certain trees in India, Malaysia and Thailand. The resin is picked from the trees by hand, purified and marketed either as orange coloured flakes, or as a bleached powder. Since it is a natural product its purity and composition vary. Shellac gives a very firm film, often slightly yellowish in colour, and tends to be brittle. It is insoluble in water but soluble in borax solution and in alcohol. A lacquer-removing shampoo containing borax or alcohol is therefore required when washing shellac-based lacquer from the hair. *The plastic resins* used in lacquers, namely PVP/VA and DMHF, are the same as described under setting lotions (see page 180).

The solvents used in lacquers are industrial methylated spirit, isopropanol or ethanol.

The main additives used to modify the film are
1. Plasticisers such as isopropyl myristate or dimethyl phthalate to soften the plastic film.
2. Cetrimide to give antistatic properties.
3. Silicones to ensure a good spread over the surface of the hair.
4. Lanolin which is added as a conditioner if the lacquer is intended for dry hair.

The formulation of lacquers

Shellac-based lacquer usually contains 8–10 per cent shellac dissolved in alcohol and is often applied from a puffer spray rather than an aerosol, as it is corrosive to metal cans. Lanolin may be added as a plasticiser.

Plastic resin lacquers contain 4–6 per cent of resin dissolved in alcohol, with additives of silicones, cetrimide and isopropyl myristate. They are often dispensed from an aerosol can with a non-flammable propellant such as dichlorodifluoromethane which reduces the fire risk since the alcohol solvent is highly flammable. Ethanol is used as the solvent in aerosols since any water present would react with the propellant, forming acids which would corrode the can.

Sun screen lacquers contain para-aminobenzoic acid added to a plastic resin-based lacquer. The para-aminobenzoic acid absorbs some of the ultra-violet radiations from sunlight, and so to some extent protects the hair from cystine linkage breakages by ultra-violet rays, which would weaken the hair and cause relaxation of permanent waves. The acid also helps to stop the bleaching action of ultra-violet rays on both natural and dyed hair.

Experiment 10.1   Examination of lacquer films.
Spray small quantities of different brands of lacquer onto a mirror or a piece of glass and allow them to dry. Note the colour of the films. Leave the test for a few days and note any tackiness of the film.

Control creams

Control creams or dressing creams are applied to the hair after setting and drying, but before dressing out. They are designed to replace the natural oils removed during shampooing, and help to preserve the set by preventing the entry of moisture into the hair shaft. They also help to keep the hair in place, add lustre to the hair due to reflection of light by the oils, and are anti-static agents.

The creams may be water-in-oil emulsions, but are more often the oil-in-water type containing a very small proportion of water, since they are applied to dry hair and must not spoil the set. The oil may be a vegetable oil such as castor oil or almond oil, but is usually mineral oil in the form of paraffin oil.

Brilliantines

Brilliantines are also added to the hair after setting and drying, or may be sprayed onto the hair after dressing is completed.
Liquid brilliantines consist of mixtures of mineral oil and castor oil with added perfume, or when designed for spraying they contain castor oil alone, dissolved in industrial methylated spirit. An oily film is left on the hair when the spirit evaporates.
Solid brilliantines contain mixtures of paraffin oil and soft paraffin thickened by paraffin wax or carnauba wax.
Modern gel type preparations are greaseless products containing water-soluble synthetic plastic resins with a plasticiser.
Clear gels are oil-in-water emulsions using either mineral or vegetable oils. The oils are dispersed in the water as sub-microscopic particles, and feel less greasy than ordinary oil-in-water emulsions.

Questions

1. Name three factors which affect the holding power of a lacquer.
2. Explain why the application of a liquid brilliantine adds lustre to the hair.
3. Name one substance used: (a) in heat-perm lotions;
    (b) in exothermic pads   (c) as a film-former in setting lotions.
4. Give one use of each of the following substances;
    (a) silicone oils;   (b) plasticisers;   (c) ascorbic acid.

5. Explain what is meant by: (a) bound water; (b) alpha-keratin; (c) beta-keratin.
6. What is meant by a cohesive set? Describe the part played by hydrogen bonds during setting.
   Explain how a hairdresser can ensure that a client's set will be long-lasting.
7. Ammonium thioglycollate is a salt which can be prepared by the process of chemical neutralisation.
   Explain this statement and discuss the difference between chemical neutralisation and the use of a 'neutraliser' in cold waving.
8. Discuss the various methods used for straightening over-curly hair, mentioning any chemical reagents which may be used.
   Describe the dangers associated with hair straightening.
9. Discuss the possible reasons for the lack of curl in the hair after cold waving.
10. Describe the chemical reactions which take place during cold perming.
    Discuss the chemical damage which may take place during perming.

Chapter 11

Hair condition and conditioning agents

One of the most important aims of hairdressing is to maintain the client's hair in the best possible condition whilst still carrying out treatments such as bleaching, straightening, permanent waving and tinting, which are desired by the client but which tend to cause hair damage. Hair is in good condition if it feels soft and smooth to the touch, has lustre, is manageable and easy to comb, has a high tensile strength and sufficient elasticity to take a good cohesive set.

The condition of hair is partly a surface effect due to the condition of the cuticle and the degree of oiliness of the surface scales, and partly an internal effect depending on the moisture content of the cortex and the state of the chemical linkages of cortical keratin.

Surface condition

When in good condition, the cuticle scales lie flat and close together to give a relatively smooth compact surface. In damaged hair some of the scales may be raised, the surface of the scales abraded and the edges chipped, producing a rough uneven surface. If severely damaged the cuticle scales may be completely destroyed, thus exposing the cortical layer.

The condition of hair often varies along the length of the hair shaft. A hair grows for between 2 and 7 years before the follicle enters telogen and the hair is ready to be shed. If it has not been cut, the hair could be by that time between 30 and 100 cm in length, and due to damage from various sources will show progressive damage or loss of cuticle from root to tip.

Near the root, the cuticle is usually smooth but even a few millimetres from the scalp the scale edges may become more jagged. Further along the hair, the edges of the scales tend to be lifted away from the surface which becomes more and more eroded towards the point of the hair. In very long hair fragments of the cuticle may have broken off, exposing the cortex, and the tip of the hair may show longitudinal splitting. In addition to being in worse condition at the tip than at the root, hair in the frontal region usually shows more surface damage than that in other areas since it is subjected to more wear and tear by brushing and combing. Any part of the hair which is constantly subjected to friction, for example by being continually pushed away from the face or which rubs on the shoulders as

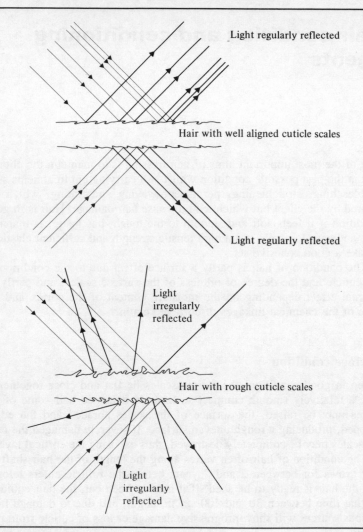

Light regularly reflected

Hair with well aligned cuticle scales

Light regularly reflected

Light irregularly reflected

Hair with rough cuticle scales

Light irregularly reflected

Fig 11.1 Light reflected from smooth and rough hair

the head turns, is likely to have poor surface condition.

Besides affecting the feel of the hair, roughness of the surface of hair leads to dullness in appearance (see Fig. 11.1).

A smooth surface reflects light regularly; that is, light leaves the surface at the same angle, which gives the surface lustre. A rough surface reflects light irregularly, so the light is diffused in all directions and the surface has a matt or dull appearance. A thin covering of oil (sebum) on the surface of the hair will increase the amount of light which is regularly reflected, so increased lustre; whereas a thick coating of oil due to over-secretion by the sebaceous glands tends to absorb light and makes hair dark and lank.

The roughness of hair, especially if it is dry, also leads to the production of static electricity when the hair is brushed or combed. This causes the hair to become positively charged. The like charges on adjacent hairs repel each other, causing fly-away hair. The brush or comb becomes negatively charged so it attracts the positive charge on the hair, which therefore follows the movement of the brush or comb. The more the hair is brushed or combed, the worse the effect becomes.

A thin coating of sebum on the cuticle makes the hair more supple and therefore less brittle. The hair is easier to comb and the danger of mechanical damage is decreased. The degreasing effect of soapless shampoos can affect the condition of hair by removing too much sebum, so allowing the moisture in the hair shaft to dry out. A general lack of sebum due to under activity of the sebaceous glands or failure to spread sebum along the hair shaft by brushing thus leads to lack of condition.

Damage to the cuticle makes the hair more porous which leads to the absorption of sebum, leaving insufficient on the surface to create lustre. Increased porosity may also lead to increased absorption of chemicals, possibly causing internal damage to the hair.

Experiment 11.1 Examination of surface damage.
Using a microscope with the highest magnification available, examine hairs from the same head before and after bleaching, to observe any surface damage. Repeat with hairs before and after perming. Using as long a hair as possible, examine the surface at intervals along its length to observe wear and tear.

Internal condition of hair

The internal condition of hair depends on the *state of the chemical linkages* in keratin and the *amount of bound water* in the hair. These factors affect both the *elasticity* and *tensile strength* of the hair.

The chemical linkages

In virgin hair the linkages formed during keratinisation are intact. Chemical treatment with strong alkalis, reducing agents or oxidising agents may damage the linkages, thus affecting the internal condition.

Alkalis with a pH of over 9.5 break the cystine linkages by hydrolysis and at a pH of 12 destroy the main polypeptide chains leading to the complete destruction of the hair.

Treatment by reducing agents such as ammonium thioglycollate will break some of the disulphide linkages but more powerful reducing agents, e.g. sodium sulphide, will also break the main polypeptide chains, so destroying the hair. Whilst mild oxidising agents will repair the disulphide linkages broken by reducing agents as in perming, stronger oxidising agents destroy the linkages by forming cysteic acid. Very strong oxidising solutions will break the main polypeptide chains, again leading to destruction of the hair.

Both reducing agents and oxidising agents make keratin more soluble, and particularly attack the twisted mass of polypeptide chains in the matrix between the cortical fibres. Treatment by these agents always results in loss of protein material from the hair.

The number of linkages in the cortex and their strength affects the elasticity and tensile strength of the hair.

Effect of water on hair

The amount of water in 'dry' hair depends on the relative humidity of the surrounding air. If the air is dry, hair will lose water to the air and when the air is humid will gain water. Hair normally contains about 15 per cent of water whilst in air of relative humidity about 70 per cent and a temperature of 20 °C (a normal room temperature). An intact cuticle and coating of sebum on the hair tends to prevent water either entering or leaving the hair shaft.

When hair is soaked with water, it is drawn into the minute spaces between the polypeptide chains by capillary action and tends to force the chains apart, causing swelling of the hair. The amount of water entering the spaces depends on the number and strength of the cross linkages which hold the chains together. In undamaged hair nearly all the swelling due to absorption of water takes place between the cortical fibres in the matrix of twisted polypeptide chains. The amount of swelling is increased if a large number of cross linkages, especially disulphide linkages, have been destroyed as in overbleaching, since a great deal of water will enter the spaces between polypeptide chains of the cortical fibres themselves. The amount of swelling when hair is soaked in water is thus a guide to the extent of damage to the cross linkages.

In addition to the 'free' water which is absorbed in the spaces between the chains, a certain amount of water becomes bound in the protein molecules, especially in the hydrogen bonds. It is this 'bound' water which increases elasticity. Some conditioners are effective by their ability to bind water to the hair. The presence of water in the hair also reduces the tendency of static electrical charges to be produced on the hair surface, since the moist hair becomes a conductor and the electricity leaks away to earth.

Experiment 11.2   To demonstrate damage to cross linkages.
Cut two small pieces of hair each about 2 cm long, from a single hair shaft. Soak one of the pieces in water for 30 minutes and then mount both pieces side by side on a microscope slide and cover with a coverslip. Compare the diameters of the two pieces of hair, measuring the diameter using a microscope scale. Repeat, using different hairs, such as a bleached hair, a recently permed hair, and a tinted hair.

Compare the diameter of the soaked hair with that of the dry corresponding hair in each case, to estimate the damage to the cross linkages.

Elasticity

Hair in good condition will stretch due to the coiled spring arrangement of its molecular structure. The extension of the hair is opposed by the presence of numerous hydrogen bonds between the polypeptide coils and by the cross linkages between adjacent polypeptide chains, and when the stretching force is removed the hair will spring back to its original length. The cuticle scales slip over each other if the hair is stretched, so do not oppose the extension. Thus, hair which is in good condition is elastic.

However, if dry hair is extended more than about 30 per cent of its original length the hair reaches its *elastic limit* or *yield point*. If extended beyond this limit the hair no longer returns to its original length when the stretching force is removed. When stretched beyond this limit, hair suddenly extends rapidly due to the breakage of the hydrogen bonds and the unfolding of the α-helix. If stretching is continued, the hair will eventually reach *breaking point*.

Hair is more elastic when wet, as the water molecules enter the hydrogen bonds to allow greater extension. If the water content of the hair is increased from the 5 per cent in 'dry' hair to 30 per cent, the percentage elongation (that is the percentage of its original length that a hair is being stretched) increases from 30 to 50 per cent before the elastic limit is reached.

Breakage of the salt linkages by weak acids or weak alkalis also permits greater extension of hair. Maximum extension is at a pH of about 5, but at pH values below 3 the ability to stretch is reduced as the water content is decreased. If the disulphide linkages are reduced in number as in chemical damage to the hair, greater extension is possible but the hair no longer springs back to its original length when the stretching force is removed. Thus the elasticity of chemically damaged hair may be considerably reduced; for example, in over-bleached hair.

Tensile strength

The strength of a hair fibre depends on the strength of the polypeptide chains in keratin and also on the cross linkages holding the chains together. The force in grammes per square millimetre (g/mm^2) required to break the hair is known as its tensile strength and is about 20 kg/mm^2 for a dry hair. An average hair in good condition will support a mass of 120–150 g before breaking. The tensile strength may vary at different points along the hair shaft and the hair will break at its weakest point. Breakage may occur across the hair by breakage of the polypeptide chains or by the molecules slipping apart from each other, causing a frayed type of break.

The tensile strength of wet hair is less than that of dry hair so that a wet hair will support less weight. Chemical damage to the disulphide linkages or to the polypeptide chains themselves weakens the hair.

Machines to measure elasticity and tensile strength of hair are available. They measure the percentage elongation at breaking point and the force in grammes required to stretch the hair to breaking point.

Experiment 11.3 Determination of the percentage elongation and breaking point of hair.

Use the apparatus as shown in Fig. 11.2 to find the percentage elongation of hair and the force in grammes required for it to reach breaking point.

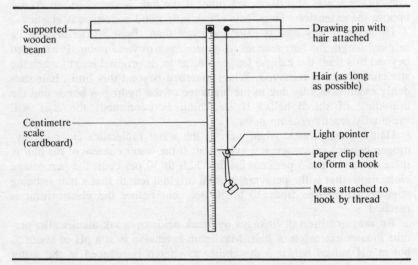

Fig 11.2 Determination of percentage elongation and breaking point of hair

Choose as long a hair as possible and measure its length. Increase the load gradually and note the length of the hair at each addition to the load. Continue until the hair breaks.

Test   1. Dry hair.
       2. Wet hair.
       3. Hair which has been soaked in dilute acetic acid.
       4. Hair which has been bleached.
       5. Hairs from the same head before and after perming.

Repeat each experiment several times using hairs from the same head, and obtain the average force at breaking point for each group. Calculate in each case the percentage elongation, i.e.

$$\frac{\text{length of hair at breaking} - \text{original length}}{\text{original length}} \times 100$$

Calculate this value in each case and hence the average for each group. Compare the averages for the groups, together with the breaking forces.

Cause of lack of condition in hair

Lack of condition may be caused by:

Internal physiological factors, including poor general health, specific diseases, the after effects of child birth, diet, drugs, the over or under activity of the sebaceous glands and excessive scalp perspiration.

External factors including chemical damage, mechanical damage and weathering.

It is with the external factors that the hairdresser has most control though treatment of lack of condition due to internal factors would also be carried out.

Causes of mechanical damage

The cuticle scales of hair can be eroded by any form of friction applied to the hair. The effect is increased if the hair is wet, as the cuticle is softened and more easily removed or damaged.

Mechanical damage to the cuticle by friction can be caused during:

1. *Excessive massage of the scalp* whilst shampooing.
2. *Towel drying.* Blotting the hair dry is less damaging than vigorous rubbing.
3. *Normal brushing and combing.* Frequent harsh brushing can abrade the cuticle especially if an unsuitable brush is used. Natural bristles taper at the tips, but in cheap nylon brushes they have cut edges which may be rough and jagged, though they may be tapered in more expensive types. Combing to remove tangles can cause the lifting of the cuticle, particularly in tightly curled hair. Broken or badly made combs may cause hair breakage.

   Bleached and permed hair, which have fewer cystine linkages than untreated hair, are particularly susceptible to mechanical damage by brushing and combing. Splitting of these hairs may take place even when the cuticle is intact.
4. *Back brushing and back combing*, which may damage the cuticle by breaking off small fragments which have become slightly raised from the surface of the hair.
5. *Brushing or combing wet hair* as in blow waving. Damage is reduced by the use of silicone setting lotions.

Once the cuticle has been removed the cortex is easily damaged especially by wet brushing. This may result in splitting of the hair shaft especially at the points.

Mechanical damage may also be caused by the use of spiked rollers or excessively tight rollers, the continual use of postiche, by combing during hair straightening processes and by tension applied to hair after reduction has taken place in cold waving. Incorrect razor cutting by use of a slithering action can strip off sections of cuticle scales up to 2 cm in length and leave areas which easily become frayed.

Causes of chemical damage

Most chemical damage takes place during the processes of bleaching, hair straightening and permanent waving (see Fig. 11.3). The possible damage is considered in detail in Chapter 9 for bleaching damage and in Chapter 10 for damage during straightening and permanent waving.

Damage to the cuticle is caused by any alkaline treatment including bleaching, hair straightening, tinting and permanent waving and the use of alkaline shampoos and setting lotions. Alkalis make the hair swell and roughen the scales of the cuticle. Sections of scales often break away during both bleaching and perming. The scales may be scorched during blow drying if the hot nozzle touches the hair.

Damage to the disulphide linkages always occurs in perming and bleaching. Reduction during perming breaks some of the linkages and fewer are replaced during subsequent oxidation so that there is always a significant loss of linkages. A greater loss occurs through over-processing or faulty neutralising. During bleaching, up to 50 per cent of the disulphide linkages may be destroyed by oxidation.

Loss of protein material also always takes place during perming and bleaching since some of the oxidation products are soluble in water.

Breakage of the hair shaft due to chemical damage to the polypeptide chains may occur by:
(a) use of products with a pH greater than 9.5, e.g. too long contact time with sodium hydroxide in hair straightening;
(b) excessive oxidation during bleaching;
(c) burning of the hair during heat setting or heat perming;
(d) use of hydrogen peroxide on hair previously treated with metallic dyes;
(e) the perming of damaged hair, e.g. excessively bleached hair.

Weathering

Weathering is the effect on hair structure of exposure to climate conditions, particularly to strong sunlight. The effect of weathering is difficult to distinguish from that of chemical and mechanical damage.

Exposure to ultra-violet rays in sunlight causes breakage of the disulphide linkages, and so may reduce the tensile strength of the hair and cause relaxation of perms. Heat from the sun dries out the hair, roughens the cuticle and encourages hair breakages and split ends. The effect of sunlight is greater if the hair has previously been damaged by cosmetic treatment – for example, bleaching – or if the hair is already weakened as in cases of monilethrix. At the end of long, hot summers there is a seasonal increase in cases of fragilitas crinium and trichorrhexis nodosa.

Sunscreen lacquers (see Chapter 10) may be used to lessen damage by sunlight but a more effective way is to cover the hair and avoid over exposure to the sun.

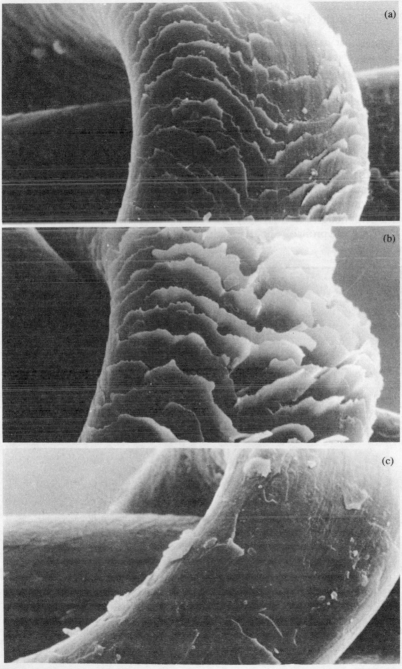

Fig 11.3 Electron micrographs of human hair showing the effect of perming and bleaching (a) untreated hair (b) hair permed 10 times (c) hair bleached 3 times

Defects in the hair shaft

Chemical or mechanical damage and weathering may result in defects of the hair shaft such as fragilitas crinium and trichorrhexis nodosa.

Fragilitas crinium (split ends or trichoptilosis)

If hair becomes very dry and brittle it often splits lengthways, usually at the ends but possibly also at various points along the shaft (see Fig. 11.4). The condition often occurs in long hair, the tips of which may have been subjected to daily brushing and combing, shampooing and possibly periodic perming, dyeing or bleaching over a number of years. The best and simplest treatment is to cut the split ends off and improve the condition of the remainder of the hair by use of cationic or protein conditioners. Split ends cannot be permanently repaired by protein conditioners though they may help the ends to cling together electrostatically. They would probably hold together equally well if hair lacquer were applied.

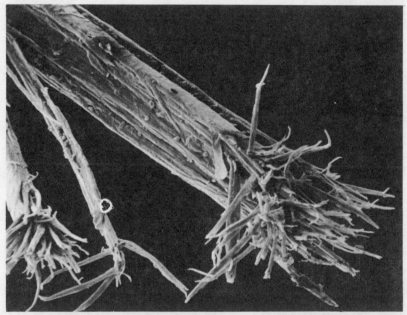

Fig 11.4 Fragilitas crinium (showing frayed structure of the split end of a hair)

Trichorrhexis nodosa

A series of *split nodes* which appear at various points on the hair shaft are characteristic of trichorrhexis nodosa (see Fig. 11.5). The hair is weak at the nodes and breakages often occur at these points. The condition may be caused by the use of spiked rollers or other mechanical means, or by strong alkalis. Seasonal trichorrhexis nodosa occurs in late summer due to

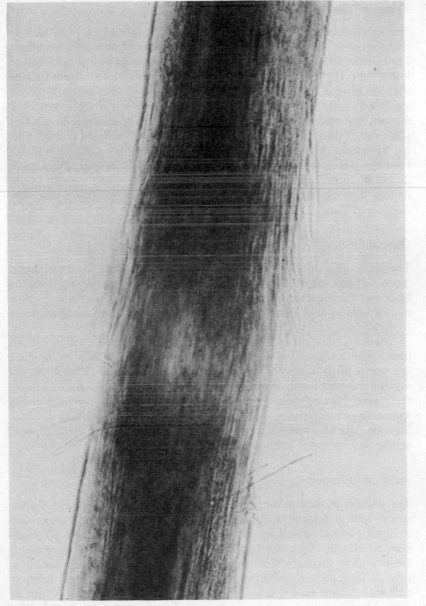

Fig 11.5 Trichorrhexis nodosa

the effect of sunlight and perhaps sea-water which causes degradation of keratin and weakening of the hair shaft. Treatment is by cetrimide or protein conditioners.

Types of conditioner

The removal of sebum during shampooing, or general lack of sebaceous secretion, was at one time thought to be the cause of poor hair condition. The earliest conditioners were therefore oily substances designed to replace lost sebum. However, if hair is completely degreased by a solvent such as trichloroethane the hair is left shiny and manageable, smooth to the touch with little tendency to develop statical electrical charges. It is now thought that poor condition is largely due to lack of moisture in the hair shaft rather than deficiency of grease. Thus many modern conditioners are humecants designed to attract water to the hair. Oils still have a place, however, since their presence on the hair helps to prevent the loss of moisture. Acids have long been used as conditioners and are still in use though their purpose has changed. Many modern conditioners are substantive to hair.

Oil conditioners

The application of oil to the hair has an emollient effect since the hair is made soft and supple. A light coating of oil reduces friction between the hairs and the brush or comb, so preventing mechanical damage. Reflection of light by the oil increases lustre. Oils also prevent loss of moisture from the hair and control wisps.

Vegetable oils such as olive oil and almond oil are used in hot oil treatments though this type of conditioning has largely been replaced by the use of sulphonated oil shampoos and cetrimide rinses. Castor oil and mineral oils are used in dressing creams and brilliantines. Lanolin and synthetic products made to resemble sebum are added as conditioners to cream shampoos, cream rinses, hair dyes, lacquers and conditioning creams. Silicone oils are being increasingly used and are added to shampoos, setting lotions, perm solutions and cream rinses.

Acid conditioners

The traditional need to use weak acids such as tartaric acid, citric acid, acetic acid and lactic acid, as rinses to remove lime soap after soap shampoos and to neutralise the alkali, no longer exists. Almost all shampoos are soapless so do not form scum in hard water and most have added citric acid to give a pH of about 6.5–7. Acids are however useful as rinses after processing with other alkaline reagents in bleaching, perming and tinting. Ascorbic acid is often used for this purpose as it is also an antioxidant and helps to stop the action of hydrogen peroxide after processing is completed. The use of acid after bleaching and perming precipitates any soluble protein material formed and so prevents its loss from the hair.

Substantive conditioners

The group of substantive conditioners includes cationic detergents, non-ionics and ampholytes, protein hydrolysates and polyvinyl pyrrolidone. They cling to the hair electrostatically and their effect remains even after rinsing and drying. Some of these substances also condition by acting as humecants or water-attracting agents, which thus help to bind extra water inside the hair shaft.

Cationic detergents such as cetrimide act as emollients, making the hair softer (they are also used as fabric softeners in laundry work), and re-peated or excessive use can over-soften the hair. Cationics reduce static electrical charges on the hair. They make the hair surface smoother so that it is easier to comb, being less tangled and therefore less liable to breakage during combing. Their main use is in conditioning rinses for use after shampooing. They are also added to setting lotions, perm lotions, lacquers and to after-bleach, after-perm and after-tint condition-ers. Damaged hair takes up more cetrimide than undamaged hair due to the increase in free acid groups in damaged hair.

Non-ionic detergents such as alkanolamides also act in much the same way as cationics but since they are compatible with anionic detergents they may also be added as conditioners to anionic detergent shampoos. Nonionics are often added to lacquers as antistatic agents.

Ampholytes are used in shampoos in the same way as non-ionics.

Polyvinyl pyrrolidone, a plastic resin, is a substantive conditioner which acts as a humecant and is added to shampoos and cold wave lotions.

Protein hydrolysates (see also Chapter 7) contain amino acids, dipep-tides and short chains of amino acids. The amino groups (basic groups) in the protein hydrolysates will cling electrostatically to any free acid groups in the hair in the same manner as the formation of salt linkages, and similarly the acid groups in the hydrolysates will cling to any free amino groups. Protein hydrolysates thus even out free groups which may have been formed during such processes as bleaching and perming. Damaged hair attracts more protein hydrolysates than undamaged hair because there are more unattached groups and also because the hair is more porous and more molecules of the hydrolysate will be small enough to enter the hair shaft. Consequently protein hydrolysates are used as conditioners in after-perm and after-bleach conditioners and in perm lotions themselves. They are most valuable when used as 'fillers' before perming and bleach-ing, to prevent loss of protein material during processing. In addition, they are added to shampoos and setting lotions. The surface of the hair is made smoother and more lustrous but any marked increase in tensile strength is doubtful.

The polarising microscope

Specially adapted polarising microscopes are used in some salons either as a projection microscope, so that the client may see samples of her own hair displayed on a screen, or fitted with a polaroid camera so that colour photographs can be quickly produced.

The colour obtained by these polarising microscopes depends on an *anisotropic substance* being viewed under *polarised light*. An anisotropic substance is one which has different physical properties in different directions. The cortex of the hair is anisotropic because it consists of long fibrils arranged parallel to the length of the hair. Its properties along the length are therefore different to those across the diameter of the hair. The keratin of the cuticle, medulla and the matrix of the cortex is not anisotropic but isotropic, because the molecules are arranged at random in a twisted mass so the properties are the same in any direction.

The light waves of polarised light travel in one plane only and not in random directions as does 'ordinary' light (see Fig. 11.6). If the view of the hair seen through a polarising microscope shows a continuous band of colour in the cortical area this indicates a regular protein structure. Any change in colour along the length of the hair may indicate an area of

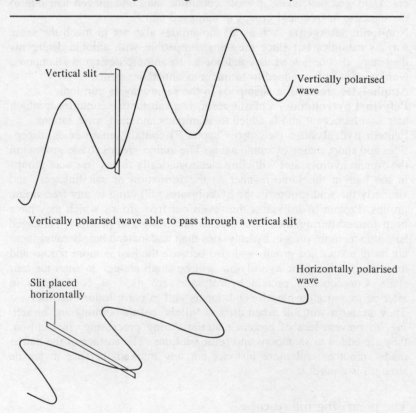

Vertical slit

Vertically polarised wave

Vertically polarised wave able to pass through a vertical slit

Horizontally polarised wave

Slit placed horizontally

Horizontally polarised wave able to pass through a horizontal slit

Fig 11.6 Polarised light

weakness in the structure. The actual colour produced depends on the diameter of the hair and on the compactness of the structure.

The use of a polarising microscope may appear dramatic to the client and it has uses in detecting and demonstrating hair damage in special cases, but its usefulness as a general guide to hair condition is somewhat limited.

Questions

1. Explain what is meant by:
   (a) a humecant;   (b) an emollient;   (c) the weathering of hair.
2. Describe the effects on hair of:
   (a) a lack of sebum;   (b) an excess of sebum.
3. Describe three ways in which hair may suffer mechanical damage.
4. Explain the advice you would give to a client who complained of:
   (a) split ends;   (b) excessively dry hair;   (c) excessively greasy hair.
5. Describe the effect on hair structure, of treatment with:
   (a) reducing agents;   (b) oxidising agents.
6. With reference to hair, explain the following terms:
   (a) tensile strength;   (b) elasticity;   (c) elastic limit;
   (d) percentage elongation.
7. Explain what is meant by 'bound' water and 'free' water in the hair shaft.
   What is the effect of bound water on the elasticity of hair?
8. Explain the various types of chemical damage which may result from:
   (a) bleaching;   (b) perming.
   Describe the general condition of hair which has been over-processed during bleaching.
9. Discuss the effect on the hair and skin of over exposure to sunlight.
10. Discuss the various uses of cetrimide in hairdressing. Describe the effect of cetrimide on the hair and explain any dangers associated with its use.

Chapter 12

Manicure

Manicure means the care of the hands including the finger nails. Many hairdressing salons offer a manicure service to their clients, which may include hand massage, the shaping of the nails and the cosmetic treatment of both skin and nails. It is important too that hairdressers themselves have attractive and well-cared-for hands, since these are important tools constantly held in view of the clients. Avoidance of contact with substances which may damage or discolour the skin and nails, the careful sterilisation of manicure tools and the correct use of cosmetic materials will help to ensure the good condition of the hands.

The anatomy of the lower arm, wrist and hand

The complicated movements of which the hand is capable depend on the bone structure of the wrist and hand, and the muscles which control the movements of these bones. There are few muscles in the hand itself and most of the muscles used in hand movements are situated in the lower

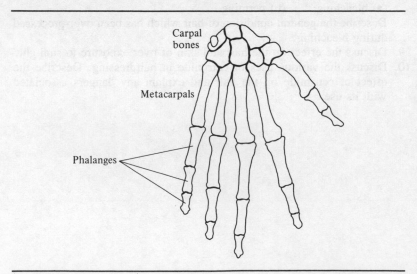

Fig 12.1 The bones of the hand and wrist

arm, being connected to the fingers by long tendons. Thus the hand is slim, and this facilitates grasping and the fine movements of which it is capable. The many small bones (eight in each wrist and nineteen in each hand), and hence the large number of joints between the bones, enables a wide range of hand movements to be performed.

The bone structure of the hand and wrist is shown and the bones named in Fig. 12.1. The wrist (or carpus) consists of a group of eight small irregularly shaped carpal bones, arranged in two rows of four with gliding joints between the two rows to allow slight movement of the wrist. The upper row forms a double hinge joint with the radius, one of the long bones of the forearm. The lower row, nearest the hand, forms gliding joints with the five metacarpal bones which run along the palm of the hand. The four metacarpals which are attached to the bones of the fingers are almost parallel to each other, whilst that attached to the base of the thumb is set at an angle, enabling the thumb to move very freely in many directions. The thumb itself consists of two short bones whilst each finger has three bones. In the thumb and fingers, the bones, called phalanges, are connected by hinge joints, allowing movement in one direction only. The rounded heads of the metacarpals form the knuckles,

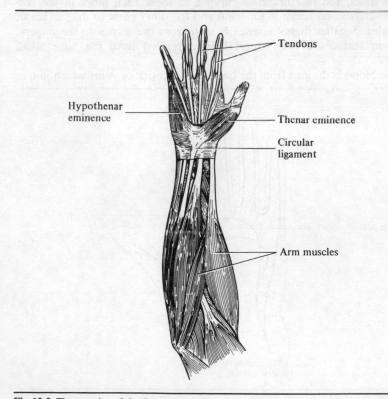

Fig 12.2 The muscles of the forearm and hand

where they articulate with the lower bone of each finger. These joints are double hinge joints and allow movement in two directions.

The muscles of the forearm and hand are shown in Fig. 12.2. The tendons which move the fingers, are attached at one end to the arm muscles and to the bones of the finger tips at the other. By placing the hand palm downwards on a flat surface and raising the fingers and thumb, the tendons along the back of the hand may be felt. These are known as the extensor tendons and are used to straighten the fingers on contraction of the appropriate arm muscle. In the palm of the hand are the flexor tendons which are used to close the fingers as in gripping an object in the palm of the hand. The tendons of the arm muscles are bound at the wrist by a circular ligament just above the wrist joint.

The muscles of the hand itself consist of a short flexor muscle for the thumb and muscles which enable the fingers to move from side to side. These are most prominent on the palm of the hand, at the base of the thumb (the thenar eminence) and at the base of the little finger (the hypothenar eminence).

The blood supply to the hand is shown in Fig. 12.3. The radial and ulnar arteries of the forearm carry blood to the hand. At the wrist each artery forks, the two branches curving to meet each other in the two palmar arches, one deep in the hand and the other close to the surface of the palm. Smaller digital arteries branch from the arches to the fingers, adjacent surfaces of the fingers being supplied from the same small artery.

The blood is drained from the hand in a network of veins which join to

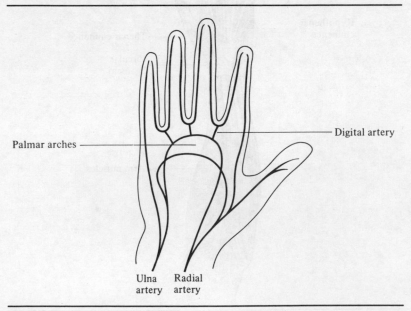

Fig 12.3 The blood supply to the hand

form the three main veins running along the forearm and taking blood back to the heart.

The skin of the hands

The palmar surface of the hand has a large number of sweat glands, more in fact than in any other area of skin except the soles of the feet. There are, however, few sebaceous glands on the palms and no vellus hairs. The stratum lucidum of the epidermis is thicker on the palms than in other areas except the soles and gives rise to the thick palmar skin. The numerous ridges on the palms and fingers are due to the large number of dermal papillae below the epidermis. These provide numerous positions for nerve endings, making the finger tips very sensitive. The ridges also afford good gripping properties, and as there is a fixed pattern of ridges for each person, 'finger prints' may be used for the identification of individuals.

The skin on the backs of the hands is quite different, being relatively thin and soft with fine vellus hairs. There are large numbers of both sweat and sebaceous glands. The nerve endings are far less numerous than on the palms and it is possible to find isolated spots which are insensitive to cold, heat or pain.

Conditions affecting the hands

Contact dermatitis

Some substances used in manicure may cause irritation of the skin, resulting in contact dermatitis. A substance affecting the skin is a primary irritant if it affects the skin on first contact, and the dermatitis is limited to the area of contact. If it causes sensitisation which is followed by an allergic reaction at any subsequent contact it is called an allergen (see also Chapter 3). The symptoms are similar in both cases and may consist of reddening of the skin with vesicles, papules and some swelling of the area. In the case of an allergic reaction the eruption is not limited to the area of contact but may also affect other parts of the skin.

Substances used in manicure which are likely to cause dermatitis include lanolin in hand creams, formaldehyde resin in nail enamel and methyl methacrylate in artificial finger nails. Dermatitis due to nail cosmetics may occur on the face rather than round the nail itself if the more sensitive skin of the face is touched by the nails. Special cosmetics are available from which all likely irritants or sensitisers are omitted.

Age spots

Large brown freckle-like spots often appear on the backs of the hands as a person ages. These are known as senile freckles, age spots or sometimes as liver-spots, though they have no connection with the liver. They are caused by exposure to the sun over a long period. Age-spots may be treated by creams containing hydroquinone but this is sometimes unsuccessful and some people become allergic to the compound. Alternatively they may be hidden by waterproof cover-up make-up. Further spots and the enlargement of existing spots can be avoided by use of a sun-protection cream during exposure to sunlight or by complete avoidance of the sun.

Chilblains

Chilblains are irritant red swellings on the fingers and are usually troublesome in the winter time. The remedy is to improve the circulation in the fingers by exercise or massage and to always keep the hands warm by wearing gloves in cold weather.

Rough skin

Patches of rough skin on the palms of the hands can be softened by the application of olive oil.

Tobacco stains

These may be removed by use of 5 vol hydrogen peroxide, or by rubbing the area with pumice stone followed by the application of hand cream.

Warts

Warts are caused by a virus infection of the epidermis. Since they are unsightly and also contagious, they should be removed by a doctor though they may eventually disappear without treatment. Warts are considered more fully in Chapter 3.

Scabies

Infestation by itch mites may result in the development of burrows which appear as short dark lines in the skin between the fingers or on the front of the wrists. Medical attention is required. See also Chapter 3.

Skin cosmetics for the hands

Hand creams

These are oil-in-water emulsions in the form of liquid or solid creams which act as emollients or skin softeners. Some of the water from the emulsion is absorbed by the epidermis but most evaporates to leave a layer of oil. This prevents loss of moisture from the skin and makes it smoother by cementing down rough surface scales. Glycerol and lanolin are often added as extra emollients. Hand creams are designed to replace sebum lost during washing.

Glycerol and rose water

Glycerol and rose water may be used as an alternative to hand cream. The product is oftened thickened by the addition of gum tragacanth. Glycerol should not be used on the skin without dilution with water, as it is a humecant and would absorb moisture from the skin, thus defeating the object of its application. Glycerol and rose water usually contains about 25 per cent of glycerol.

Barrier creams

Barrier creams are oil-in-water emulsions with a vanishing cream base. Their water-repellent properties are due to the addition of silicone fluids.

Massage creams

These are oil-in-water emulsions containing liquid paraffin and olive oil with borax and beeswax as the emulsifying agent. Massage creams should be applied to the skin of the hands once or twice a week and the hand massaged, starting at the finger tips and working along the fingers, then over the palms and backs of the hands. This improves the blood circulation to the skin, softens the skin and helps to prevent chilblains.

Sunscreen creams

The most efficient sunscreen creams contain opaque substances such as zinc oxide or titanium dioxide which cut off all the sun's rays. Covering the skin with clothing is however more effective. Other sun-blocking preparations contain para-aminobenzoic acid to filter out the most damaging of ultra-violet rays but to allow through the rays which cause tanning.

The structure of the nails

Nails are protective structures made of hard keratin with a low moisture content. They grow from the germinating layer of the epidermis in a similar way to the growth of hair. The structure of a growing nail is shown in section in Fig. 12.4.

The nail plate itself consists of
1. *The root* which lies under the nail fold or cuticle.
2. *The nail body* which forms the main part of the nail.
3. *The lunula* or half moon which is an area of incomplete keratinisation

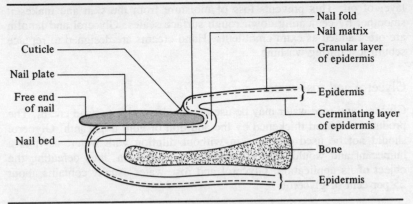

Cuticle

Nail plate

Free end of nail

Nail bed

Nail fold

Nail matrix

Granular layer of epidermis

Epidermis

Germinating layer of epidermis

Bone

Epidermis

Fig 12.4 Section through the end of a finger to show nail growth

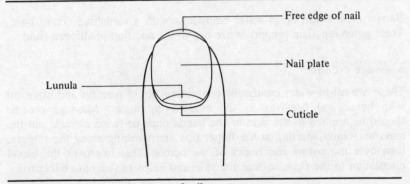

Free edge of nail

Nail plate

Lunula

Cuticle

Fig 12.5 End of finger to show parts of nail

and is held by loose connective tissue to the nail bed.

4. *The projecting or free edge* of the nail which extends beyond the end of the finger and is detached from the skin (see Fig. 12.5).

As it grows the nail moves along furrows or nail grooves at the sides of the nails and is protected by the folds of skin or nail walls, which overlap the sides and base of the nail body. The granular layer of the epidermis is absent under the nail plate except in the area of the lunula, so the nail plate rests on and is firmly attached to the cells of the prickle cell layer. The nail plate is translucent but appears pink due to the blood vessels in the dermis below. The nail cuticle is part of the horny layer of the epidermis and extends on to the nail plate at the base of the nail. Its function is to prevent infection reaching the nail matrix.

The growth of the nails

Nails are identifiable in the embryo at the third month. Growth is continuous and takes place by division of cells in the nail matrix, which is part of the germinating layer of the epidermis. The nail bed is also thought to play a part in nail formation. The cells are pushed forwards by the production of new cells. In the matrix the cells are soft but they lose their nuclei, become flattened parallel to the nail surface and are hardened by keratinisation. The cells lose their identity to form a mass of hard keratin. The interlocking of keratin fibrils gives a compact structure to the nails.

The nail bed and the matrix are well supplied by blood vessels which bring nutrients and oxygen to the growing nail. The rate of growth of finger nails is 2.5 mm a month and is slightly faster than toe nails. Since ultra-violet rays stimulate cell division, growth is slightly faster in summer than in winter. The rate of growth decreases with age and in some illnesses, especially if fever is present. In cases of psoriasis growth is quicker than normal, particularly if thimble-pitting is a symptom. Complete regrowth if a nail is lost takes about 5½ months.

Defects of the nails

Many nail defects are caused by internal physiological conditions such as anaemia and psoriasis but some are due to mechanical trauma. Occasionally nails may be congenitally absent.

Paronychia

Paronychia means inflammation of the tissue round the nail. It may be caused by damage to the cuticle especially if incompletely sterilised manicure tools are used. An abcess or whitlow results and the nail plate may be damaged or even shed. The area becomes red, swollen and tender. Manicuring should be avoided until healing is complete.

Onycholysis

The separation of the nail plate from the nail bed is known as onycholysis. It may be caused by an accident or as a result of ringworm infection, psoriasis, or dermatitis of the finger tips.

Ringworm of the nail

This fungal infection causes the nail to crumble and become yellow and powdery at the base and sides of the nail (see Fig. 12.6). The condition can be cured by taking the drug griseofulvin orally. The drug becomes attached to newly formed keratin and so protects it from infection. The affected part of the nail can be cut off as it grows. No manicure service should be given and if a client is thought to have ringworm of the nail medical attention should be advised.

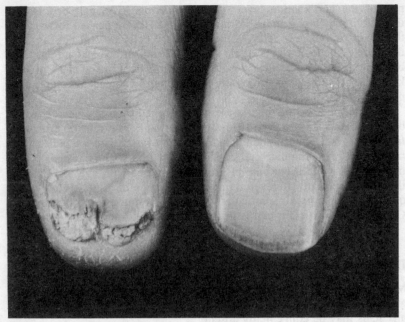

Fig 12.6 Ringworm of the nail

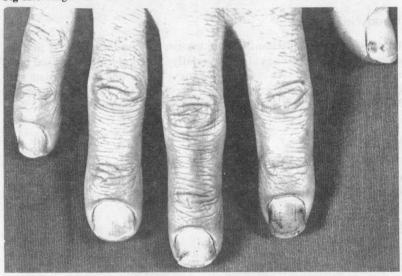

Fig 12.7 Psoriasis causing thimble pitting of the finger nail

Psoriais of the nails

Psoriasis often, but not necessarily, results in the thimble pitting of the nails as well as the formation of large silvery scales on the scalp and elbows (see Fig. 12.7). Scales may also form at the nail fold, on the nail bed or under the free edge of the nail. Medical attention is required.

Fragilitas unguium (brittle nails)

The normal 18 per cent water content of nails keeps them flexible. Dehydration of the nail leads to brittle nails, which easily split or break at the free edge. The condition is often caused by the frequent use of detergents or of solvents such as acetone or amyl acetate in nail enamel and enamel remover. This results in loss of water by removal of the protective barrier of oil from the skin and nail. Brittle nails are often associated with iron deficiency anaemia.

Frequent immersion of the hands in water should be avoided and the use of rubber gloves is advised. Fragile nails can be artificially strengthened by use of nail enamel containing nylon fibres.

The eating of gelatin (table-jelly cubes) is often said to improve brittle nails but there is no scientific evidence to support the idea. The protein in gelatin is broken down during digestion like all other proteins and used along with amino acids from all other foods for general body building and repair. Gelatin is in fact deficient in certain essential amino acids.

Soft nails

Nails are softened by constant immersion in water and by contact with alkalis. Cold wave lotions soften nails in the same way as keratin is softened during perming. The condition can be avoided by the use of rubber gloves.

Discoloration of nails

The yellowing of nails may be due to smoking, the taking of various drugs, staining by nail enamel pigment or the effect of ringworm fungus. The darkening of nails takes place on contact with chemicals such as potassium permanganate, silver nitrate and para dyes, or may be the result of conditions such as psoriasis and contact dermatitis. Black areas under the nails are caused when bleeding takes place between the nail itself and the nail bed. This may be due to mechanical damage to the nail, for example, if the finger ends have been trapped. The discoloration eventually grows out.

White spots on the nails are caused by injury to the matrix or damage to the body of the nail resulting in the separation of a portion of of the plate from the nail bed. There is no remedy and the spots eventually grow out. The whole nail becomes white if it is detached from the nail bed.

Mis-shapen nails

Koilonychia (spoon-shaped nails)
This condition often occurs in middle aged women due to iron deficiency

anaemia or to lack of cystine in the nail structure. The nails have concave surfaces and are thin and soft.

Hang nails

These are the result of the splitting of narrow strips of nail along the nail groove. They may be the result of dry nails or to damage during manicure.

Grooving

This may consist of either vertical or horizontal ridges on the nail. Vertical ridges are hereditary, though they tend to show more with age which could indicate dryness. Horizontal ridges (Beau's lines) often run across the nails of both hands and indicates some past illness such as measles or pneumonia in which there was a temporary cessation of growth of all the nails. If only one nail is affected it may be due to damage to the matrix, perhaps due to inflammation of the base of the nail.

Nail cosmetics

The main products used on the nails are cuticle removers, cuticle creams, nail enamels, nail lacquer removers and nail hardeners.

Cuticle remover

If the cuticle encroaches too far over the nail plate it may be removed by use of a 2 per cent solution of either sodium hydroxide or potassium hydroxide. These are caustic alkalis which soften keratin and dissolve it. Sebum from the cuticle and nail area will be removed at the same time, so the use of cuticle remover tends to dry the nail and surrounding skin. Excess cuticle remover should be rinsed off with water, followed by the application of cuticle cream or an emollient containing glycerol. Sometimes glycerol is added to the cuticle remover itself to counteract the de-greasing effect.

Cuticle massage cream or milk

Cuticle creams or milks are water-in-oil emulsions containing mineral oils and water, with borax and beeswax as the emulsifying agent. Glycerol may be added as an emollient. The proportion of oil is greater in creams than in milks, and creams are thus more suitable for use if the cuticle skin is dry and the nails brittle.

Nail white pencil

The whiteness of the projecting nail may be increased by applying nail white pencil under the free edge of the nail when a clear nail enamel is to be used. The material is a soap base containing a white pigment such as titanium dioxide.

Paste polish (buffing powder)

The effect of buffing is to increase the circulation to the nail area and give shine to the nail. Buffing is carried out using a chamois leather pad and a buffing powder containing talc or kaolin and stannic oxide. If a nail enamel is to be used, buffing before application of the enamel produces a smooth base for the application.

Nail enamel (nail lacquer or varnish)

Nail enamel is designed to enhance the appearance of the nails by the application of a tough glossy film, either coloured or transparent. The film should adhere firmly to the nail, be resistant to abrasion, chipping or peeling, and resistant also to water, detergents and other chemicals with which the enamel may come into contact. The colour should be fast to light, and should not stain the nail or surrounding skin. The enamel should be easy to apply and form an even film with no brushmarks. It should be sufficiently viscous so that it does not run off the nail during application, but should be quick drying and should form a long-lasting hard film with a high gloss.

Enamel is basically a solution consisting of the *film-former* (the solute) which carries the colour, dissolved in a *solvent* with suitable drying properties. The properties may be modified by additions such as *plasticisers* to soften the film, colour and perfume. On application to the nail the solvent evaporates, leaving the film adhering to the nail.

The film-former is usually a mixture of nitro cellulose and synthetic resins such as formaldehyde resin. Used by itself nitro cellulose has poor adhesion, is brittle and lacks gloss. The addition of synthetic resins improves these qualities, helping the enamel to stick to the nail.

The solvent is a blend of volatile substances to give the correct rate of drying. If the solvent evaporates too quickly the enamel thickens and does not flow easily so that brush marks are left in the final film. The rapid evaporation may cause sufficient cooling of the nail so that moisture from the air condenses on its surface, resulting in a cloudy film. If less volatile solvents are used, drying may be inconveniently slow. A suitable solvent consists of mixtures of ethyl acetate, butyl acetate and toluene. Acetone is now rarely used as it increases the tendency to cloud.

To improve the flexibility of the film and prevent chipping and cracking of the film on the nail, plasticisers are added, usually in the form of esters such as dibutyl phthalate or isopropyl myristate or sometimes glycerol.

The pigment may be synthetic or may be a mixture of such substances as iron oxide, chromium oxide, titanium dioxide, carbon black and ultramarine. The colour must not fade or react with other substances in the enamel. Pearl effects are obtained by the addition of natural pearl essence obtained from fish scales, usually herring, and containing crystals of guanine which reflect light at various depths in the enamel. Synthetic crystals in the form of highly reflective platelets of bismuth oxychloride may also be used.

The addition of up to 0.1 per cent of silicone oil improves the appearance and adhesive properties of nail enamel. If 0.5–1 per cent of silicones is used, the oil heightens the gloss and protects the enamel against water and detergents.

At least two coats of enamel are applied. The first or base coat is designed to key the enamel to the nail and prevent chipping of the film. It is less viscous than the top coat and gives a thinner film. Base coats also contain a lower percentage of film-former. When the base coat is dry the top coat is applied to give a thicker film which is usually coloured and has a high gloss.

Nail enamels are flammable and must be kept away from heat sources and flames. To avoid fading of colouring matter, they should be stored out of sunlight in a cool dark place. When not in actual use the bottle should be stoppered to avoid evaporation of the solvents. Otherwise the most volatile of the solvents in the mixture would evaporate first and upset the balance of the solvents. If by careless use nail enamel dries out either wholly or partially, it may be impossible to renew the correct blend of solvents. Addition of nail enamel remover may help to liquidise the enamel but will not restore the blend.

Nail enamel remover

Liquid types of enamel remover contain a mixture of solvents which will re-dissolve the enamel from the nail. These include amyl acetate, butyl acetate or ethyl acetate with an added emollient such as castor oil to counteract the drying effect of the solvents, and leave a thin film of oil on the nail after the enamel is removed. Acetone is now rarely used as a solvent in enamel remover as it is considered to be too de-greasing to the nail and skin.

Cream enamel removers are emulsions containing nonionic emulsifying waxes and a low percentage of water, with triethanolamine soap as the emulsifying agent. The emulsion also contains about 60 per cent of solvents such as amyl acetate or butyl acetate to re-dissolve the enamel film. Cream removers are less de-greasing than liquid types.

Nail hardeners

Nail hardeners are designed to prevent the chipping or peeling of nails and consist of formaldehyde resins. Since the resin is a potential sensitiser and many people are allergic to it, the skin round the nail and the cuticle should be protected by oil before application of the resin. Allergic reaction to the resin may result in swelling of the skin around the nail, discolouration of the nail or loss of the nail plate.

Artificial finger nails

1. Some artificial finger nails are formed on the nails themselves by painting a plastic polymer on the nail. The polymer consists of methyl methacrylate along with a hardener. The two are mixed just before use and brushed over the nail as a thick liquid. The polymer hardens quickly at room temperature and becomes firmly attached to the nail, eventually growing out with the nail.

   The polymer may cause contact dermatitis, the skin adjacent to the nail becoming inflamed and swollen, and in severe cases the nail may be detached from the nail bed. It is difficult to treat because the artificial nail cannot be removed, and takes several months to grow out.

2. False nails may be attached to the natural nail by adhesives, the artificial nail merely being pressed into position and filed to the shape of the nail. This type of nail should not be left in position for more than a few days since the natural nail becomes softened underneath the plastic nail.

Nail menders

Nail menders contain film-formers of nitro-cellulose and formaldehyde resin, with a reinforcing material consisting of short rayon or nylon fibres. The resins are dissolved in a solvent of ethyl acetate, the fibres being held suspended in the solution by addition of a silica gelling agent. A plasticiser is added and the solution may be coloured. The mender is applied in four coats, each being applied at right angles to the previous coat, the film being allowed to dry between the applications.

Questions

1. What are the beneficial effects of massage of the hands?
2. Explain the function of:
   (a) the nail grooves;   (b) the nail matrix.
3. Describe how the nails could be affected in cases of:
   (a) psoriasis;   (b) ringworm;   (c) anaemia.
4. What are the symptoms of contact dermatitis caused by an allergy to nail enamel?
5. State three possible reasons for discoloration of the nails.
6. Discuss the variations in the skin of different parts of the hands. What precautions should a hairdresser take to keep her own hands in good condition?
7. What is the function of the cuticle of the nail?
   Name the main ingredients of cuticle remover.

What dangers may result from damage to the cuticle during manicuring or by the misuse of cuticle remover?

8. What are the qualities of a good nail enamel?
   How does this affect the choice of materials used during manufacture?

9. Discuss the advice you would give to a client who complained of:
   (a) vertical grooving of the nails;   (b) brittle nails;   (c) short dark lines appearing in the skin between the fingers;   (d) swelling and inflammation of the skin round the nails;   (e) yellowing of the nails.

10. Discuss the meaning of
    (a) Beau's lines;   (b) hang nails;   (c) paronychia;   (d) the palmar arches;   (e) the nail bed.

Multiple choice questions

In the following questions, choose in each case the most suitable answer from the four possible alternatives given.

Chapter 1

1 The zygomatic arch joins the zygomatic bone to the

(a) occipital bone
(b) sphenoid bone
(c) parietal bone
(d) temporal bone

2 The squamosal suture lies between

(a) the two parietal bones
(b) the frontal and parietal bones
(c) the occipital and parietal bones
(d) the parietal and temporal bones

3 The areas of fibrous tissue between the bones of an infant's skull are called

(a) fontanelles
(b) foramina
(c) sinuses
(d) sutures

4 The three main branches of the external carotid artery are the

(a) ophthalmic, mandibular and maxillary
(b) facial, temporal and ophthalmic
(c) cervical, occipital and temporal
(d) occipital, temporal and facial

5 A sensory nerve carries information

(a) from the brain to the skin
(b) down the spinal cord
(c) from a sense organ to the brain
(d) from the brain to a sense organ

6 The three branches of the trigeminal nerve are

(a) maxillary, zygomatic and temporal
(b) mandibular, temporal and cervical
(c) buccal, temporal and ophthalmic
(d) maxillary, mandibular and ophthalmic

7 The cranial nerve carrying information to the brain from the skin of the face is called the

(a) trigeminal
(b) facial
(c) abducent
(d) accessory

8 Which of the following are muscles of mastication?

(a) risorius and platysma
(b) orbicularis oris and oculi
(c) temporalis and masseter
(d) frontal and zygomatic

9 The muscles causing frowning are the

(a) frontalis
(b) buccinators
(c) sternomastoids
(d) corrugator supercilii

10 Nutrients and oxygen are carried from the capillaries to the living cells of the body by

(a) lymph
(b) blood plasma
(c) tissue fluid
(d) arterial blood

Chapter 2

1 Exposure to ultra-violet rays may cause
   (a) increased secretion of perspiration
   (b) erythema of the skin
   (c) suppression of sebaceous secretion
   (d) an increase in hair loss

2 The production of sebum is controlled by
   (a) hormones
   (b) nerve stimulation
   (c) contraction of the hair muscles
   (d) enzymes

3 The sebaceous glands are
   (a) endocrine glands
   (b) eccrine glands
   (c) holocrine glands
   (d) apocrine glands

4 The nerve endings in a Meissner's corpuscle are sensitive to
   (a) cold
   (b) heat
   (c) pain
   (d) touch

5 The phagocytic cells of the dermis are
   (a) scavenger cells
   (b) secretory cells
   (c) oxygen-carrying cells
   (d) pigment producing cells

6 The epidermis
   (a) has a good blood supply
   (b) obtains nourishment from the blood vessels of the dermis
   (c) is dead tissue so does not have a supply of blood
   (d) has blood vessels only in the lower layers

7 Glabrous skin contains
   (a) no sebaceous glands
   (b) no hair follicles
   (c) an excessive number of follicles
   (d) an excessive number of sweat glands

8 Erythema means
   (a) redness of the skin
   (b) massage of the scalp
   (c) exposure to ultra-violet rays
   (d) heat treatment by infra-red rays

9 Freckles are caused by a
   (a) localised concentration of pigment in the lower dermis
   (b) concentration of pigment on the surface of the skin
   (c) a large group of melanocytes in the lower epidermis
   (d) a congenital growth

10 The stratum corneum of the epidermis is
   (a) a layer of actively dividing cells
   (b) the protective layer of the skin
   (c) the layer containing most pigment
   (d) composed of living keratin

Chapter 3

1 Hyperidrosis describes a condition of excessive
   (a) hair growth
   (b) hair loss
   (c) secretion of sebum
   (d) production of sweat

2 Wood's light is used
   (a) for the treatment of warts
   (b) to improve salon lighting
   (c) to detect ringworm fungus
   (d) to improve the circulation of blood to the scalp

3 The electromagnetic rays produced by Wood's light are
   (a) infra-red rays
   (b) X-rays
   (c) rays of pure white light
   (d) ultra-violet rays

4 Ringworm fungus obtains nourishment from the skin by
   (a) digesting keratin by enzyme action
   (b) sucking blood from the dermis
   (c) burrowing into the dermis
   (d) absorbing sweat and sebum from the surface of the skin

5 Folliculitis refers to
   (a) infestation by face mites
   (b) ingrowing hairs in the beard area
   (c) a predisposition to boils
   (d) inflammation of the hair follicles

6 Head lice may be destroyed by treatment with

(a) cetrimide
(b) griseofulvin
(c) malathion
(d) acetic acid

7 The 'bottle bacilli' associated with dandruff are

(a) bacteria
(b) enzymes
(c) viruses
(d) yeasts

8 The active ingredient in modern antidandruff shampoos is

(a) acetic acid
(b) zinc pyrithione
(c) benzylbenzoate
(d) formaldehyde

9 Which of the following is caused by a virus infection?

(a) warts
(b) moles
(c) milia
(d) impetigo

10 Psoriasis is caused by

(a) a virus infection
(b) damage to the germinating layer
(c) faulty production of keratin
(d) reaction to ultra-violet rays

Chapter 4

1 A hair follicle is said to be in telogen when

(a) the follicle is resting
(b) the hair is actively growing
(c) the follicle is changing to the resting stage
(d) a new hair is beginning to grow in the follicle

2 Huxley's layer is part of the

(a) hair shaft
(b) inner root sheath
(c) outer root sheath
(d) dermis

3 A bulge which appears on the side of the developing follicle in the foetus

(a) forms a point of attachment for the arrector pili muscle

(b) forms the area from which the arrector pili muscle grows
(c) becomes the inner root sheath
(d) becomes the hair papilla

4 Glabrous skin is found on the

(a) backs of the hands
(b) soles of the feet
(c) forehead
(d) under the chin

5 The function of Henle's layer of the inner root sheath is to

(a) hold the hair securely in the follicle
(b) enable the inner root sheath to slip easily over the outer root sheath
(c) connect the inner and outer root sheaths firmly together
(d) to pass melanin into the cortex

6 Hairs are sensitive to touch due to the

(a) presence of the arrector pili muscle
(b) the nerve fibres in the papilla
(c) collar of nerves round the follicle
(d) nerve endings in the hair shaft itself

7 The zone of keratinisation of hair in the follicle is

(a) in the inner root sheath
(b) in the germinal matrix
(c) at the base of the follicle
(d) above the level of the bulb

8 Peptide linkages form part of

(a) polypeptide chains
(b) disulphide bonds
(c) amino acids
(d) ionic bonds

9 In the hair cortex several polypeptide chains twisted together form

(a) a salt linkage
(b) an alpha-helix
(c) an amino acid
(d) a protofibril

10 The matrix between cortical fibres consists of

(a) actively dividing cells
(b) protofibrils
(c) cystine linkages
(d) twisted polypeptide chains

Chapter 5

1 Nutrients reach the dividing cells of
the hair matrix by means of

   (a) tissue fluid
   (b) tissue respiration
   (c) lymph ducts
   (d) blood which bathes the cells

2 Severe lack of protein in the diet may
result in a condition known as

   (a) kwashiorkor
   (b) anaemia
   (c) rickets
   (d) fragilitas crinium

3 Deficiency of vitamin C in the diet
may lead to

   (a) small bald patches on the scalp
   (b) accumulation of scale in the
       follicles
   (c) haemorrhages round the hair
       follicles
   (d) a reduction in the period of
       anagen

4 Which of the following is an
endocrine gland?

   (a) sebaceous gland
   (b) thyroid gland
   (c) lachrymal gland
   (d) suderiferous gland

5 During pregnancy, changes in
hormone levels may cause

   (a) an increase in the period of
       anagen
   (b) diffuse hair loss at about the 6th
       month
   (c) many follicles to enter the resting
       stage
   (d) an increase in the rate of hair
       growth

6 Hyperaemia refers to

   (a) reddening of the skin
   (b) increase in blood flow to the area
   (c) excessive hair growth
   (d) excessive perspiration

7 The massage action given by the use
of the spiked rubber applicator of a
vibro-massage machine is
   (a) petrissage
   (b) effleurage
   (c) percussion
   (d) tapotement

8 Which of the following conditions is
contraindicative of massage?

   (a) dermatitis
   (b) pityriasis
   (c) alopecia
   (d) hyperidrosis

9 The intended effect of high frequency
treatment is to

   (a) stimulate nerve endings
   (b) stimulate muscle action
   (c) produce hyperaemia
   (d) produce erythema

10 Excess intake of vitamin A in the diet
causes

   (a) increased secretion of sebum
   (b) diffuse hair loss
   (c) bald patches on the scalp
   (d) increased rate of hair growth

Chapter 6

1 Which of the following is associated
with the development of alopecia
areata?

   (a) club hairs
   (b) lanugo hairs
   (c) exclamation mark hairs
   (d) knotted hairs

2 Trichonodosis refers to hair which is

   (a) split at the ends
   (b) knotted close to the scalp
   (c) twisted along its length
   (d) fragile at its nodes

3 During electrolysis, hair is removed
by

   (a) heat produced by an electric
       current
   (b) sodium chloride in the tissues
   (c) the production of sodium
       hydroxide
   (d) an alternating current

4 Hypotrichosis refers to

   (a) excessive growth of the hair
   (b) excessive secretion of sweat
   (c) diffuse hair loss
   (d) sparseness of scalp hair

5 'Epilation' means

(a) the removal of the hair shaft
(b) destruction of the hair follicle
(c) removal of hair shaft and hair root
(d) removal of hair by electrolysis

6 Chemical depilatories may contain

(a) hydrogen peroxide
(b) calcium thioglycollate
(c) triethanolamine
(d) selenium sulphide

7 During hair removal by electrolysis, bubbles of gas rise in the follicle. This gas is

(a) air
(b) hydrogen
(c) oxygen
(d) nitrogen

8 During diathermy, hair is removed from the follicle by

(a) heat
(b) ionisation
(c) sodium hydroxide
(d) high voltage supply

9 Which of the following conditions is due to faulty pigmentation of hair?

(a) monilethrix
(b) trichonodosis
(c) leucotrichosis
(d) pili torti

10 Diffuse hair loss may be caused by

(a) an illness involving high fever
(b) constant 'twiddling' of a lock of hair
(c) repeatedly dressing the hair in a pony tail
(d) an excessive exposure to X-rays

Chapter 7

1 A substance which is 'substantive to hair' is one which

(a) increases tensile strength
(b) may be substituted for sebum
(c) clings to acid groups in the hair
(d) has strong antiseptic properties

2 The amount of cetrimide in hairdressing preparations should be limited to 2 per cent because cetrimide is

(a) damaging to the eyes
(b) a caustic substance
(c) a strong reducing agent
(d) strongly acidic

3 Which of the following substances is substantive to hair?

(a) hydrogen peroxide
(b) lanolin
(c) cetrimide
(d) sodium lauryl sulphate

4 A chemical depilatory containing calcium thioglycollate would have a pH value of about

(a) 2
(b) 7
(c) 9.5
(d) 12

5 A 9 per cent solution of hydrogen peroxide has the same strength as one of

(a) 10 vol
(b) 20 vol
(c) 30 vol
(d) 40 vol

6 An essential oil is

(a) a volatile oil obtained from plants
(b) an animal secretion
(c) a form of lanolin
(d) a volatile mineral oil

7 The 'acid mantle' of the skin has a pH of approximately

(a) 3
(b) 5.5
(c) 9.5
(d) 14

8 To prepare a '1 part in 10 solution' from a shampoo concentrate, add to each 1 part of concentrate

(a) 9 parts of water
(b) 9 ml of water
(c) 10 parts of water
(d) 10 ml of water

9 To prepare 30 ml of 6 per cent hydrogen peroxide solution from an 18 per cent stock solution, use

(a) 10 ml of 18 per cent hydrogen peroxide and 20 ml of water
(b) 20 ml of 18 per cent hydrogen peroxide and 10 ml of water

(c)   18 ml of 18 per cent hydrogen peroxide and 12 ml of water

(d)   6 ml of 18 per cent hydrogen peroxide and 24 ml of water

10 Silicone oils are used in heat setting lotions to

(a)   transmit the heat to the hair
(b)   protect the hair during drying
(c)   hold the hair in the desired position
(d)   replace sebum

Chapter 8

1 The term 'hydrophobic' means

(a)   water hating
(b)   water loving
(c)   easily dissolved in water
(d)   absorbing water

2 Soap is

(a)   a hydroxide
(b)   an anionic detergent
(c)   a cationic detergent
(d)   a non-ionic surfactant

3 Which of the following soaps would have the lowest pH value?

(a)   potassium palmitate
(b)   potassium oleate
(c)   sodium stearate
(d)   triethanolamine oleate

4 Which of the following substances is incompatible with a sodium lauryl sulphate shampoo?

(a)   cetrimide
(b)   lauryl diethanolamide
(c)   lauryl betaine
(d)   triethanolamine lauryl sulphate

5 Which of the following substances is a cationic detergent?

(a)   cetyl trimethyl ammonium bromide
(b)   triethanolamine lauryl sulphate
(c)   ammonium thioglycollate
(d)   lauryl diethanolamine

6 An ion is

(a)   an electrically charged atom or group of atoms
(b)   a hydrophobic group
(c)   a type of detergent
(d)   a surface active agent

7 Soapless detergent shampoos are often preferred to soap shampoos because they

(a)   do not degrease the hair as much
(b)   usually have a higher pH value
(c)   are more substantive to hair
(d)   do not form a scum with hard water

8 Which of the following substances may be used as a foam booster in triethanolamine lauryl sulphate shampoos?

(a)   Turkey red oil
(b)   lauryl diethanolamide
(c)   triethanolamine
(d)   cetrimide

9 A soapless shampoo designed for greasy hair may contain

(a)   extra lanolin
(b)   an increased amount of detergent
(c)   a strong antiseptic
(d)   cetrimide

10 Which of the following substances is both a detergent and a good antiseptic?

(a)   hexachlorophane
(b)   zinc pyrithione
(c)   cetrimide
(d)   sulphonated castor oil

Chapter 9

1 Loss of natural hair colour during ageing may be due to

(a)   failure by the body to produce the enzyme tyrosinase
(b)   a lack of melanocytes
(c)   oxidation of melanin by exposure to the air
(d)   genetic failure to produce melanin

2 Bleach boosters may contain

(a)   nascent oxygen
(b)   magnesium carbonate
(c)   ammonium persulphate
(d)   polyphosphates

3 The yellowing of bleached hair may be caused by

(a)   application of olive oil as a conditioner

(b) use of a cetrimide conditioner
(c) lack of exposure to sunlight
(d) use of plastic resin lacquers

4 Methyl violet is

(a) a cationic dye
(b) an oxidation dye
(c) an acid dye
(d) an azo dye

5 If auburn hair is viewed in blue light it would appear

(a) blue
(b) purple
(c) black
(d) red

6 Which of the following substances may be added during manufacture to prevent premature oxidation of permanent tints?

(a) benzyl alcohol
(b) ammonium hydroxide
(c) urea peroxide
(d) sodium sulphite

7 Ascorbic acid is used in after-bleach treatments because it

(a) is substantive to hair
(b) is both an acid and an oxidising agent
(c) is both an acid and a reducing agent
(d) neutralises any hydrogen peroxide left on the hair

8 Unwanted orange shades developed during hair colouring may be corrected by adding a little

(a) blue dye
(b) green dye
(c) red dye
(d) yellow dye

9 Melanin is formed by the oxidation of

(a) keratin
(b) tyrosine
(c) pheomelanin
(d) cystine

10 Which of the following substances is often used as an antioxidant after using a permanent dye?

(a) ascorbic acid
(b) amino acid
(c) salicylic acid
(d) phosphoric acid

Chapter 10

1 The chemical process taking place in heat perming is mostly one of

(a) oxidation
(b) reduction
(c) hydrolysis
(d) polymerisation

2 The heat set obtained by Marcel waving is due to changes in

(a) the disulphide bonding
(b) hydrogen bonding
(c) salt linkages
(d) peptide linkages

3 The process of reduction in cold waving involves

(a) changing cysteine to cystine
(b) the removal of hydrogen bonds
(c) taking oxygen from the hair
(d) adding hydrogen to the sulphur atoms of cystine linkages

4 Which of the following substances is effective as a hair straightener?

(a) calcium oxide
(b) sodium stearate
(c) zinc pyrithione
(d) ammonium thioglycollate

5 The ability of hair to stretch depends on

(a) the coiled polypeptide chains
(b) the presence of the hydrogen bonds
(c) the strength of the disulphide linkages
(d) the electrostatic attraction of the salt linkages

6 Wet hair will stretch more than dry hair because

(a) the disulphide linkages are weakened
(b) water lubricates the hair
(c) water molecules enter the hydrogen bonds
(d) the electrical charge on the hair is reduced

7 Oil-in-water emulsions are often preferred to water-in-oil emulsions used as control creams since they

(a) are easily washed from the hair
(b) are more stable
(c) contain a higher proportion of oil
(d) form a thicker cream

8 Plasticisers are added to plastic lacquers to

(a)   coat the hair with a plastic film
(b)   soften the hair shaft
(c)   soften the plastic film
(d)   make the lacquer longer lasting

9 Permed hair always suffers chemical damage because
(a)   the hair is over-stretched during perming
(b)   there is less sebum on the cuticle
(c)   not all the disulphide linkages are reformed
(d)   the hydrogen bonds contain more water

10 A disulphide group is present in

(a)   a cysteine linkage
(b)   a cystine linkage
(c)   a lanthionine linkage
(d)   a peptide linkage

Chapter 11

1 A hair in good condition has lustre because its relatively smooth surface

(a)   reflects light regularly
(b)   diffuses the light
(c)   disperses the light
(d)   absorbs the light

2 Over-bleached hair will absorb a lot of water because

(a)   there are fewer cross-linkages between the chains
(b)   the air spaces between the chains are narrower
(c)   there are more hydrogen bonds in damaged hair
(d)   the keratin has become dried out

3 The yield point of a hair is the stage at which

(a)   the hair breaks
(b)   the alpha-helices of keratin rapidly begin to unfold
(c)   the hair starts to stretch
(d)   the tensile strength is greatest

4 Over-exposure of hair to ultra-violet rays, e.g. sunlight, may lead to

(a)   relaxation of perms due to breakage of cystine linkages

(b)   a decrease in the rate of growth of hair
(c)   improvement in the condition of the hair
(d)   damage to the hair by the breakage of the polypeptide chains

5 'Protein fillers' contain

(a)   plastic polymers
(b)   a high percentage of protein
(c)   amino acids and peptides
(d)   synthetic resins

6 Fly-away hair is caused by

(a)   the degreasing action of shampoos
(b)   static electrical charges on the hair
(c)   insufficient grooming
(d)   over-vigorous towel drying after shampooing

7 Humecant hair conditioners

(a)   attract water which becomes 'bound' to the hair
(b)   prevent the entry of water into the hair
(c)   soften the cuticle scales
(d)   leave a film of oil over the hair surface

8 The tensile strength of hair depends largely on

(a)   the percentage of protein in hair
(b)   the amount of bound water in the hair
(c)   the strength of the polypeptide chains
(d)   the number of hydrogen bonds in the hair

9 Hair which has been bleached is weakened due to

(a)   oxidation of disulphide linkages
(b)   removal of pigment granules
(c)   reduction of disulphide linkages
(d)   over-stretching the cuticle

10 Trichoptilosis refers to

(a)   hair with split ends
(b)   a type of ringworm
(c)   very fragile hair
(d)   chemically damaged hair

Chapter 12

1 The number of bones in a hand and a wrist together is

(a) 8
(b) 19
(c) 27
(d) 28

2 The term 'onycholysis' refers to

(a) inflammation of the nail fold
(b) separation of the nail plate from the nail bed
(c) brittle nails
(d) mis-shapen nails

3 Which of the following substances may be used as a solvent for nail enamels?

(a) water
(b) formaldehyde resin
(c) ethyl acetate
(d) glycerol

4 Nails grow from

(a) dermal tissue
(b) the lunula
(c) the nail fold
(d) epidermal tissue

5 The joints between the bones of the wrist are

(a) hinge joints
(b) gliding joints
(c) fixed joints
(d) ball and socket joints

6 Pure glycerol should not be applied to the hands as it is

(a) an emollient
(b) a humecant
(c) a depilatory
(d) a caustic substance

7 White spots on the nails may be due to

(a) a type of ringworm
(b) over use of nail enamel
(c) injury to the matrix
(d) dehydration of the nail

8 Silicone fluid may be added to nail enamels

(a) as an antiseptic
(b) to soften the enamel
(c) to add extra colour
(d) to impart gloss

9 Thimble pitting of the nails may occur in cases of

(a) ringworm of the nail
(b) psoriasis
(c) anaemia
(d) contact dermatitis

10 Spoon-shaped nails may be due to

(a) a recent feverish illness
(b) a hereditary condition
(c) iron deficiency anaemia
(d) incorrect manicure

Index